Mayo Clinic on Managing Diabetes

Maria Collazo-Clavell, M.D.

Editor in Chief

Mayo Clinic

Rochester, Minnesota

Mayo Clinic on Managing Diabetes provides reliable, practical, easy-to-understand information on controlling diabetes and preventing complications of the disease. Much of this information comes directly from the experience of endocrinologists and other health care professionals at Mayo Clinic. This book supplements the advice of your physician, whom you should consult for individual medical problems. *Mayo Clinic on Managing Diabetes* does not endorse any company or product. MAYO, MAYO CLINIC, MAYO CLINIC HEALTH INFORMATION and the Mayo triple-shield logo are marks of Mayo Foundation for Medical Education and Research.

Distributed to the book trade by Kensington Publishing Corp., New York, N.Y.

Photo credits: Cover photos and the photos on pages 1 and 97 are from PhotoDisc. Photos on pages 37 and 139 are from Stockbyte.

Library of Congress Catalog Card Number: 00-134265

ISBN 1-893005-06-2

Printed in the United States of America

First Edition

1 2 3 4 5 6 7 8 9 10

About Diabetes

More Americans than ever before have diabetes. The disease affects an estimated 16 million adults and children. That's approximately 6 percent of the population, or 1 in every 17 people. What's more, only about half of the people with diabetes have their disease under control. This is unfortunate because researchers continue to identify methods to better manage this common illness. Unlike years ago, today if you receive a diagnosis of diabetes, you have a good chance of living an active and healthy life — provided you and your doctor take the necessary steps to control your blood sugar (glucose).

Within these pages you'll find practical advice you can use to successfully manage your diabetes and reduce your risk of serious complications. If you're at risk of the disease, you'll learn about lifestyle changes that may keep you from developing diabetes. This book is based on the expertise of Mayo Clinic doctors and the advice they give day in and day out in caring for their patients.

About Mayo Clinic

Mayo Clinic evolved from the frontier practice of Dr. William Worrall Mayo, and the partnership of his two sons, William J. and Charles H. Mayo, in the early 1900s. Pressed by the demands of their busy surgical practice in Rochester, Minn., the Mayo brothers invited other physicians to join them, pioneering the private group practice of medicine. Today, with more than 2,000 physicians and scientists at its three major locations in Rochester, Minn., Jacksonville, Fla., and Scottsdale, Ariz., Mayo Clinic is dedicated to providing comprehensive diagnoses, accurate answers and effective treatments.

With this depth of medical knowledge, experience and expertise, Mayo Clinic occupies an unparalleled position as a health information resource. Since 1983, Mayo Clinic has published reliable health information for millions of consumers through award-winning newsletters, books and online services. Revenue from the publishing activities supports Mayo Clinic programs, including medical education and research.

Editorial Staff

Editor in Chief
Maria Collazo-Clavell, M.D.

Managing Editor
Karen R. Wallevand

Copy Editor
Mary Duerson

Editorial Researchers
Deirdre A. Herman
Shawna L. O'Reilly

Contributing Writers
Lee J. Engfer
Rebecca Gonzalez-Campoy
Tamara Kuhn
Stephen M. Miller

Creative Director
Daniel W. Brevick

Layout and Production Artist
Craig R. King

Graphic and Medical Illustrators
Brian S. Fyffe
John Hutcheson
Craig R. King
Michael A. King
M. Alice McKinney
James D. Postier
Christopher P. Srnka

Editorial Assistant
Carol A. Olson

Indexer
Larry Harrison

Reviewers and Additional Contributors

Elaine M. Eisenman, R.N.
Donald D. Hensrud, M.D.
Frank P. Kennedy, M.D.
Yogish C. Kudva, M.D.
Michael A. Morrey, Ph.D.
Roger L. Nelson, M.D.

Robert A. Rizza, M.D.
F. John Service, M.D.
Steven A. Smith, M.D.
Carol L. Willett, R.D.
Bruce R. Zimmerman, M.D.

Preface

If you're reading this book, chances are you or someone close to you has diabetes or is at risk of getting the disease. You may not be sure what this means. Should you worry? Should you expect big changes in your life? Should you fear what your future holds?

Diabetes is a serious — and increasingly common — illness. But no longer is it a disease shrouded in uncertainty. Today, more than ever, doctors are aware of what it takes to control diabetes to help you live a healthy and productive life. However, your doctor can't do it alone. Successful management of diabetes requires teamwork and a lifelong commitment.

In this book, we provide practical advice to help you keep your health in check. This same advice also can prevent development of diabetes if you're at risk. We'll help you understand what diabetes is and how it can affect your health if it's not well controlled. We discuss factors that are essential for controlling the disease — monitoring your blood sugar, eating a healthy diet, getting daily exercise and maintaining a healthy weight. We review various medications available for controlling diabetes, as well as advances in drug management and experimental therapies that show promise. We'll also tell you what to expect from your health care team and how to play an active role in maintaining your health and well-being.

Think of your health as your most valuable asset. Just as you wouldn't take chances on your other assets — your money, property and family — why take a chance on your health? Along with the advice of your doctor, this book can help you feel assured that you're doing the right things to manage your diabetes and reduce your risk of serious complications.

Maria Collazo-Clavell, M.D.
Editor in Chief

Contents

Part 3: Medical Therapies

Part 4: Living Well

Part 1

The Facts

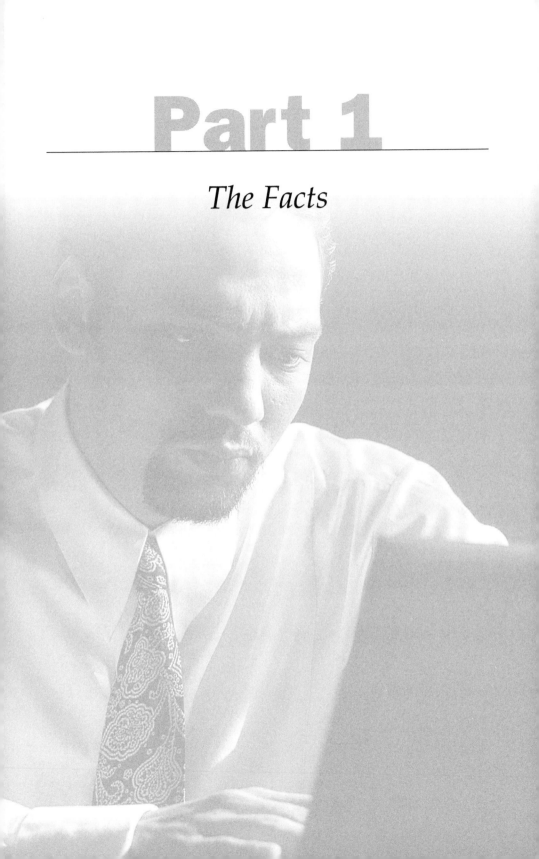

Chapter 1

Understanding diabetes

Perhaps your doctor recently broke the news that you have diabetes. Or you've learned that you're at risk of getting the disease. You're worried — afraid of what diabetes will do to you. Will you have to eat tasteless food that has no sugar? Will you have to give yourself daily shots of insulin? Will you eventually face an amputation? Will your diabetes kill you?

For the majority of people with diabetes, the answer to these questions is no. Researchers have learned a great deal about how to diagnose diabetes early and how to control it. Because of these advances, you can live well and not suffer serious complications if you follow your doctor's advice regarding eating, exercise, blood sugar monitoring and, when necessary, use of medications.

Due largely to the aging of the American population and the growing number of Americans who are overweight, diabetes has become one of the most common diseases in the United States. As your age and weight increase, so does your risk of diabetes. It's estimated that 16 million American adults and children have diabetes. Unfortunately, close to one-third don't know it. The reason: Diabetes can develop gradually over many years and often without symptoms.

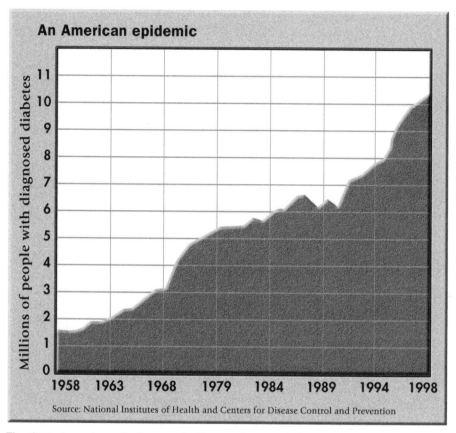

An American epidemic

Millions of people with diagnosed diabetes

11 10 9 8 7 6 5 4 3 2 1 0

1958 1963 1968 1979 1984 1989 1994 1998

Source: National Institutes of Health and Centers for Disease Control and Prevention

The chart above shows the increase in diagnosed cases of diabetes during the past 40 years. Millions more Americans are thought to have diabetes but haven't yet been diagnosed.

Left untreated, diabetes can damage almost every major organ in your body. The disease also can be fatal. Diabetes is the cause of nearly 200,000 deaths in the United States each year. That's why it's important to treat the disease as soon as you discover you have it. Lifestyle changes and medication can help you avoid or reduce complications of diabetes. Lifestyle changes also can prevent diabetes if you're at risk of the disease.

Diabetes is a serious illness, but it can be controlled. If you're willing to do your part, you can continue to enjoy an active and healthy life, despite your disease.

What is diabetes?

Understanding how your body normally handles sugar will help you to understand what diabetes is and how it occurs.

Sugar in your blood, called glucose, comes from two major sources: the food you eat and your liver. During digestion, sugar is absorbed into your bloodstream from food particles in your stomach and small intestine. This sugar is vital to your health because it's the main source of energy for individual cells that make up your muscles and tissues. However, to do its job, glucose requires a companion called insulin. The hormone insulin comes from tiny cells in your pancreas called beta cells. These cells reside in isolated masses of tissue called islets (EYE-lets). When you eat, your pancreas responds by secreting insulin into your bloodstream. As it circulates, insulin acts like a key, unlocking microscopic doors that allow sugar to enter your cells. By allowing sugar into your cells, insulin lowers the amount of sugar in your bloodstream and prevents it from reaching high levels. As your blood sugar level drops, so does the secretion of insulin from your pancreas.

Your liver, meanwhile, acts as a glucose storage and manufacturing center. When the level of insulin in your blood is high, such as after a meal, your liver stores extra sugar in case your cells need it later. When insulin levels in your blood are low, such as when you haven't eaten in a while, your liver converts the stored sugar (glycogen) into glucose and releases it into your bloodstream to keep your blood sugar level within a narrow and safe range.

In addition to insulin, several other hormones affect your blood sugar level — but in the opposite manner. In certain circumstances, hormones such as glucagon, epinephrine and cortisol counteract the effects of insulin, preventing glucose from entering your cells. The hormones also encourage your liver to release its stored sugar. As a result, your body is continuously coordinating the effects of all of these hormones to keep your blood sugar within a normal range.

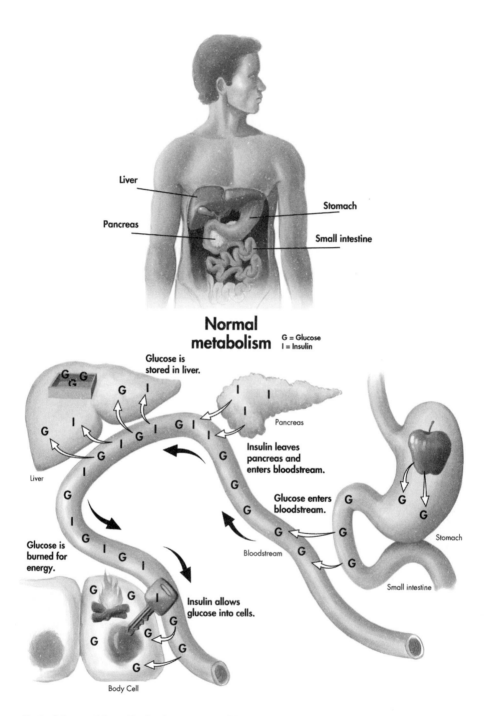

Sugar (glucose) from the food you eat provides energy to fuel your brain and body. Insulin, released by your pancreas, escorts glucose to your individual cells, where it is needed for energy, and to your liver, where extra sugar is stored.

In people with diabetes, this precisely balanced process runs afoul. Instead of being transported into your cells, glucose remains in your bloodstream, accumulates and eventually is excreted in your urine. This most often occurs for one of two reasons: Your pancreas is unable to produce insulin or your cells are unresponsive to insulin's effects.

The medical term for this condition is diabetes mellitus. Mellitus is a Latin word meaning "honey sweet," referring to excess sugar in your blood and urine. Another form of diabetes, called diabetes insipidus, is much less common. Rather than an insulin problem, it results from a hormone disorder that causes your body to lose control of its water balance, producing increased urination and excessive thirst. When we use the term diabetes in this book, we are referring to diabetes mellitus.

How much sugar is too much?

The amount of sugar in your blood naturally fluctuates, but within a narrow range. Following an overnight fast, most people have levels between 70 and 110 milligrams of glucose per deciliter of blood (mg/dL). This concentration — equal to about 1 teaspoon of sugar in a gallon of water — is considered normal.

If your blood sugar is consistently 126 mg/dL or higher after fasting, you have diabetes. At one time, a diagnosis of diabetes required a blood sugar level of 140 mg/dL or higher. The standard was lowered in 1997 after a committee of the American Diabetes Association (ADA) reviewed the results of 15 years of diabetes research. The committee found that by the time blood sugar reaches 140 mg/dL, some people already have organ damage. The ADA concluded it's best to diagnose and treat diabetes earlier, before complications develop.

If your blood sugar level measures between 111 and 125 mg/dL, you have impaired fasting glucose, commonly referred to as borderline diabetes or prediabetes. Like diabetes, borderline diabetes shouldn't be taken lightly. It's a sign that you're at high risk of developing the disease and that you should see your doctor regularly and take steps to control your blood sugar.

Types of diabetes

People often think of diabetes as one disease. But sugar can accumulate in your blood for various reasons, resulting in various types of diabetes.

Type 1

Type 1 diabetes develops when your pancreas makes little if any insulin. Without insulin circulating in your bloodstream, sugar can't get into your cells, so it remains in your blood.

Type 1 diabetes used to be referred to as insulin-dependent diabetes or juvenile diabetes. That's because the disease most often develops when you're a child or a teen, and you need to administer insulin medication daily to make up for the insulin your body doesn't produce. The names insulin-dependent diabetes and juvenile diabetes are used less often today because they're not entirely accurate. Though less common, adults also can develop type 1 diabetes — not just juveniles. In addition, use of insulin isn't limited only to people with type 1 disease. People with other forms of diabetes also may need insulin.

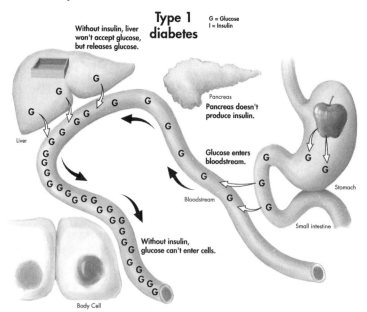

Type 1 diabetes

G = Glucose
I = Insulin

Without insulin, liver won't accept glucose, but releases glucose.

Pancreas
Pancreas doesn't produce insulin.

Glucose enters bloodstream.

Liver

Bloodstream

Stomach

Small intestine

Without insulin, glucose can't enter cells.

Body Cell

In type 1 diabetes, your pancreas produces little if any insulin. Without insulin to escort sugar (glucose) from the food you eat into your cells, glucose remains in your bloodstream.

Type 1 diabetes is an autoimmune disease, meaning that your own immune system is the culprit. Similar to how it attacks invading viruses or bacteria, your body's infection-fighting system attacks your pancreas, zeroing in on your beta cells, which produce insulin. Researchers aren't certain what causes your immune system to fight your own body, but they believe genetic factors, exposure to certain viruses and diet may be involved. The attack can dramatically reduce — even entirely wipe out — the insulin-making capacity of your pancreas.

Between 5 percent to 10 percent of people with diabetes have type 1, with the disease occurring equally among males and females. Type 1 diabetes can smolder and remain undetected for several years. More often, though, symptoms come on quickly, commonly following an illness.

Type 2

Type 2 diabetes is by far the most common form. Ninety percent to 95 percent of people beyond age 20 who have diabetes have type 2. Like type 1 diabetes, type 2 used to be called by a couple of other names: noninsulin-dependent diabetes and adult-onset diabetes. These names reflect that many people with type 2 diabetes don't need insulin shots and that the disease usually develops in adults. Similar to type 1, the names aren't entirely accurate. Children and teenagers, as well as adults, can develop type 2 disease. In fact, the incidence of type 2 diabetes in adolescents is increasing. In addition, some people with type 2 disease need insulin to control their blood sugar.

Unlike type 1 diabetes, type 2 disease isn't an autoimmune disease. With type 2 diabetes, your pancreas makes at least some insulin, but one or two other problems develop:

- Your pancreas doesn't make enough insulin.
- Your muscle and tissue cells become resistant to the insulin.

When your cells develop a resistance to insulin, they refuse to accept insulin as the key that unlocks the door for sugar. As a result sugar stays in your bloodstream and accumulates. Exactly why the

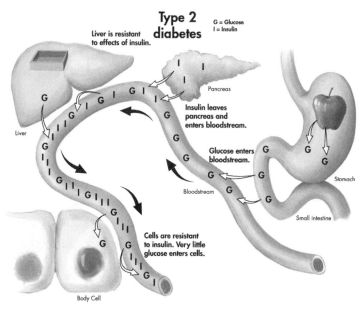

In type 2 diabetes, your pancreas produces insulin, but your cells don't respond to insulin's effects, causing glucose to remain in your bloodstream after you eat.

cells become resistant to insulin is uncertain, although excess weight and fatty tissue seem to be important factors. Most people who develop type 2 diabetes are overweight.

Over time some people with type 2 diabetes need more insulin than their pancreases can supply. Like people with type 1 diabetes, they become dependent on insulin medication to control their blood sugar.

Gestational

Gestational diabetes is the name for diabetes that develops during pregnancy. Diabetes can develop temporarily when hormones secreted during pregnancy increase your body's resistance to insulin. This happens in about 2 percent to 5 percent of pregnant women.

Gestational diabetes typically develops during the second half of pregnancy — especially in the third trimester — and usually goes away after the baby is born. But more than half of all women who experience gestational diabetes develop type 2 diabetes later in life.

Most pregnant women are screened for gestational diabetes to catch the condition early, in case it occurs. If you develop gestational diabetes, being aware of your condition and controlling your blood sugar level throughout the remainder of your pregnancy can reduce complications to you and your baby.

Other

Approximately 1 percent to 2 percent of all diagnosed cases of diabetes result from illnesses or medications that can interfere with the production of insulin or its action. They include:

- Inflammation of the pancreas (pancreatitis)
- Pancreas removal
- Adrenal or pituitary gland disorders
- Hydrocortisone treatments for another disease
- Certain high blood pressure and cholesterol-lowering medications
- Malnutrition
- Infection

Signs and symptoms

Like many people, you may have been shocked to learn that you have diabetes because you weren't experiencing any symptoms. You felt fine. Often there are no early symptoms to recognize. That's especially true with type 2 diabetes. Lack of symptoms and the slow emergence of the disease are the main reasons type 2 diabetes often goes undetected for years.

When symptoms do develop from persistently high blood sugar, they vary. Two classic symptoms that occur in most people with the disease are increased thirst and a frequent need to urinate.

Excessive thirst and increased urination. When you have high levels of sugar in your blood, your kidneys can't reabsorb all of the filtered sugar. The circulating sugar carries water with it, which is drawn from your tissues. As a result you feel dehydrated.

Diabetes warning signs

If you have diabetes you may develop any of the following signs or symptoms:

- Excessive thirst
- Frequent urination
- Hunger
- Unexplained weight loss or gain
- Flulike symptoms, including weakness and fatigue
- Blurred vision
- Irritability
- Slow-healing cuts or bruises
- Tingling or loss of feeling in hands or feet
- Recurring infections of gum or skin
- Recurring vaginal or bladder infections

To replenish the fluids being drawn out, you're almost constantly drinking water or other beverages. This water-intensive filtering process leads to more frequent urination.

Flulike feeling. Symptoms of diabetes can mimic a viral illness — fatigue, weakness and loss of appetite. Sugar is your body's main fuel. When you have diabetes, sugar doesn't get to your cells, where it's converted into an energy source. As a result you feel constantly tired or exhausted.

Weight loss or gain. As your body struggles to compensate for constant dehydration and loss of sugar, you may eat more than usual and gain weight. In other people the opposite occurs. Muscle tissues don't get enough glucose to generate growth and energy. As a result you can lose weight even though you're eating more than normal. This is especially true if you have type 1 diabetes, when little or no insulin is available and little or no sugar gets to your tissue cells.

Blurred vision. Excessive sugar in your blood pulls the fluid out of the lenses in your eyes, causing them to thin and affecting their ability to focus. Lowering your blood sugar will restore fluid to your lenses. Your vision may remain blurry for a while as your lenses adjust to the restoration of fluid. But in time your vision will improve.

High blood sugar also can cause the formation of tiny blood vessels in your eyes that can bleed. The blood vessels themselves don't produce symptoms, but bleeding from the vessels can cause dark spots, flashing lights, rings around lights and even blindness. Because diabetes-related eye changes often don't produce symptoms, it's important that you see an eye specialist (ophthalmologist or optometrist) regularly. By dilating your pupils, an eye specialist is able to examine the blood vessels in each retina.

Slow-healing sores or frequent infections. High levels of blood sugar block your body's natural healing process and its ability to fight off infections. For women, bladder and vaginal infections are especially common.

Tingling feet and hands. Excessive sugar in your blood can damage your nerves, which are nourished by your blood. Nerve damage can produce a number of symptoms. The most common nerve-related symptoms are a tingling feeling and a loss of sensation that occurs mainly in your feet and hands. This results from damage to your sensory nerves. You may also experience pain in your extremities — legs, feet, arms and hands — including burning pain. Damage to the nerves that control digestion can lead to nausea, diarrhea or constipation. Among men, diabetes can damage the nerves that help produce an erection, leading to impotence.

Red, swollen and tender gums. Diabetes may weaken your mouth's ability to fight germs, increasing your risk of infection in your gums and the bones that hold your teeth in place. Other signs of gum disease include:

- Gums that have pulled away from your teeth, exposing more of your teeth or even part of the root
- Sores or pockets of pus in your gums
- Permanent teeth becoming loose

- Changes in the fit of your dentures

Other signs. Diabetes may cause dry, itchy skin and recurring skin infections.

Factors that increase your risk

Perhaps you've heard some of the common myths about diabetes — that you can catch it from someone else, or that it comes from eating too much sugar. Not true. Researchers don't fully understand why some people develop the disease and others don't. It's clear though that your lifestyle and certain health conditions can increase your risk.

Family history. Your chance of developing either type 1 or type 2 diabetes increases if someone in your immediate family has the disease, whether that person is a parent, brother or sister. It's clear that genetics play a role in the disease, but exactly how certain genes may cause diabetes is still unknown.

Scientists are looking for genes that may be associated with type 1 and type 2 diabetes. In fact, they have found some genetic markers for type 1 diabetes, which means it's possible to screen relatives of people with type 1 diabetes to see if they also are at risk of the disease. In a study sponsored by the National Institute of Diabetes and Digestive and Kidney Diseases, relatives at risk of type 1 diabetes are being treated with low doses of either insulin or an oral medication to see if the drugs may prevent the disease.

Weight. Being overweight is one of the most obvious risk factors for diabetes. More than 8 out of 10 people with type 2 diabetes are overweight. A recent study sponsored by the Centers for Disease Control and Prevention found that among Americans who are obese, 13.5 percent have diabetes, compared with 3.5 percent of Americans at a normal weight.

The more fatty tissue you have, the more resistant your muscle and tissue cells become to your own insulin. This is especially true if your excess weight is concentrated around your abdomen. It's as though fat somehow blocks insulin from unlocking your cells to let the sugar inside.

Many people with diabetes who are overweight often can improve their blood sugar simply by losing weight. In some cases that's all it takes to bring their blood sugar back into a normal range. Even small weight loss can have beneficial effects, reducing blood sugar levels or allowing diabetes medications to work better.

Inactivity. The less active you are, the greater your risk of developing diabetes. Physical activity helps you control your weight, uses up blood sugar as energy, makes cells more sensitive to insulin, increases blood flow and improves circulation in even the smallest blood vessels. It may decrease your risk of developing type 2 diabetes by up to 50 percent.

Another advantage of exercise is that it adds muscle mass. Normally, between 70 percent to 90 percent of your blood sugar is absorbed into your muscles. A reduction of muscle mass — which commonly takes place as you grow older or as you become less physically active — can

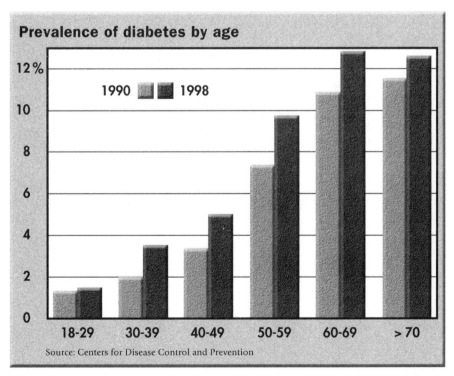

Between the years 1990 and 1998, diagnosed cases of diabetes increased within all age groups, especially young adults. The prevalence of diabetes increased nearly 70 percent among people in their 30s and approximately 40 percent among people in their 40s.

severely reduce the available storage space for blood sugar. With nowhere to go, sugar remains in your bloodstream.

Age. Your risk of type 2 diabetes increases as you grow older, especially beyond the age of 45. Nearly 1 in 5 Americans age 65 or older have diabetes. Part of the reason is that as people grow older, they tend to become less physically active, lose muscle mass and gain weight.

Recent years, however, have seen a dramatic rise in diabetes among people in their 30s and 40s. And although the prevalence of type 1 diabetes has remained steady, more children and teenagers are being diagnosed with type 2 diabetes.

Race. Though it's unclear why, people of certain races are more likely to develop diabetes than others. Approximately 6 percent of the general population in this country has diagnosed diabetes. But that rate doubles for blacks and Hispanics. And it more than doubles for American Indians, more than 12 percent of whom have diabetes. In some tribes, such as the Pima Indians, half of all adults have type 2 diabetes. Type 1 diabetes, on the other hand, is more common in whites than in blacks or other minority groups. It's also more common in European countries, such as Finland and Sweden. The reason for this is unclear.

Reducing your risk

There's nothing that you can do to avoid some of the situations in life that put you at risk of diabetes. You can't go back in time and pick a different family, different genes or a different race. And as much as you might wish that you could stop getting older, your body will continue to age. But you can control two risk factors for diabetes: weight and inactivity. And if you do, you may greatly reduce your chance of developing diabetes, especially type 2 disease.

Tests to detect diabetes

Many people first learn they have diabetes through blood tests done for another condition or as part of a routine physical examination. Sometimes, though, a doctor may test specifically for diabetes if he or she suspects the disease based on symptoms or risk factors. Any one of several tests can tell whether you have diabetes.

Finger-prick blood sugar screening

Screening tests are fast, easy and inexpensive. In fact, many health fairs offer them for free. For this reason, a lot of people are first alerted to diabetes by way of these screening tests. A finger-prick test, which usually takes no more than a couple of minutes, often requires no more than a single drop of blood from a tiny prick in your fingertip. The blood sample is placed on a chemically treated strip, which is inserted into a small machine that determines and displays your blood sugar level. If the result is above 126 mg/dL, you should have a more formal diagnostic test, such as the fasting blood sugar test.

Random blood sugar test

This test is part of routine blood work done during a physical exam. By way of a needle inserted into a vein, blood is drawn for a variety of laboratory tests. This is done without any special preparation on your part, such as an overnight fast.

Even if you've recently eaten and your blood sugar is at its peak, the level shouldn't be above 200 mg/dL. If it is, your doctor will want to confirm the results by doing a fasting blood sugar test another day.

Fasting blood sugar test

Your blood sugar level is typically highest after a meal and lowest after an overnight fast. The preferred way to test your blood sugar is after you've fasted overnight, or for at least 8 hours. Blood is drawn from a vein and sent to a laboratory for evaluation.

Most people have a fasting blood sugar level between 70 and 110 mg/dL. If your blood sugar measures 126 mg/dL or higher, your doctor may repeat the test. If your blood sugar is very high, a second test may not be necessary to reach a diagnosis. When a second test is ordered, if the results again are 126 mg/dL or higher, you'll likely be diagnosed with diabetes.

The ADA recommends that everyone have a fasting blood sugar test at age 45. If the results are normal, you should be tested every 3 years. If you have borderline diabetes — 111 to 125 mg/dL — you should have a fasting blood sugar test at least once a year. Most doctors don't screen for diabetes during routine visits, though they generally request a fasting or random blood sugar test as part of a more comprehensive examination.

Glucose tolerance test

This test is less commonly used today because other tests are less expensive and easier to administer. A glucose tolerance test requires that you visit a lab or your doctor's office after at least an 8-hour fast. There you drink about 8 ounces of a sweet liquid that contains a lot of sugar — about 75 grams. That's about three times sweeter than a soft drink.

Your blood sugar is measured before you drink the liquid, then again every hour for a 3-hour period. If you have diabetes, your blood sugar rises more than expected. If your blood sugar at the 2-hour blood test reaches between 140 and 199 mg/dL, you have a condition called impaired fasting glucose (IFG), another name for borderline diabetes. If your blood sugar at the 2-hour blood test is 200 mg/dL or above, you have diabetes.

For this test to be accurate, you should follow your usual diet and be in good health with no other illness — not even a cold. You also should be relatively active and not taking medication that could affect your blood sugar level. Doctors often use this test to check pregnant women for gestational diabetes.

Urine test

When your body isn't able to store blood sugar adequately, the excess sugar eventually is deposited in your urine. High sugar levels in urine are an indication you have diabetes. A urine test, however, generally isn't used to diagnose diabetes. One reason is that blood tests are more accurate. Also, the level of blood sugar needed to produce sugar in your urine varies from one person to another. You could have high blood sugar without sugar in your urine.

Glycated hemoglobin test

After you've been diagnosed with diabetes, your doctor may order a blood test that can measure your average blood sugar level over the previous 2 to 3 months. This gives your doctor an idea of how high your blood sugar has been in recent months, compared to other tests that measure your blood sugar level only at that immediate moment.

When your blood sugar level is high, some sugar attaches itself to oxygen-carrying hemoglobin molecules in your blood, and remains there for the life of the cell — about 2 or 3 months. The higher your blood sugar, the more hemoglobin molecules that get saddled with sugar.

A glycated hemoglobin test simply measures the amount of sugar attached to hemoglobin molecules. This test, also called the hemoglobin A-1C test, is most commonly used to monitor treatment for diabetes. You can read more about this test in Chapter 10.

Questions and answers

Is there a cure for diabetes?
No. Researchers continue looking for ways to prevent and cure diabetes, but now doctors can only treat the disease, not cure it.

How long do most people have diabetes before it's diagnosed?
Because type 1 diabetes generally occurs more suddenly and severely, it's usually diagnosed within a few months. People with type 2 diabetes, however, have the disease an average of 8 years before it's diagnosed. Regular visits to your doctor that include a complete blood workup can help prevent the disease from going undetected for so long.

Is a fasting blood sugar test always included in blood work ordered by a doctor?
No. You may have to request it. During a routine physical exam, you may have a random blood sugar test, which isn't as sensitive as a fasting blood sugar test.

What's hyperglycemia?
It's the medical term for blood sugar that's above normal — 111 mg/dL or above.

If I have a close relative with diabetes — a parent, brother or sister — what are my chances of developing the disease?
For reasons that aren't well understood, your risk of developing diabetes varies depending on whether your mother or father has or had diabetes. The table below indicates your odds for developing diabetes based on family history.

	Relative with diabetes	Your risk of diabetes
TYPE 2	Mother	19%
	Father	14%
	Both parents	25%
	Sister or brother	75%
	Twin sister or brother	99%
TYPE 1	Mother	2%
	Father	9%
	Sister or brother	10%
	Twin sister or brother	50%

Chapter 2

The dangers of
uncontrolled diabetes

D iabetes is often easy to ignore, especially in the early stages. You're feeling fine. Your body seems to be working right. No symptoms. No problem. Right?

Not even close. While you're doing nothing, the excessive sugar (glucose) in your blood is constantly eroding the very fabric of your body, threatening many major organs, including your heart, nerves, eyes and kidneys. You may not feel the effects right away, but you will eventually.

When you have diabetes you're:

- Twenty times more likely to develop kidney disease

- Four times more likely to have a stroke

- Four times more likely to become blind

- Two to four times more likely to have a heart attack

Researchers continue to make great progress in understanding what triggers complications of diabetes and how to manage or prevent them. Several long-term studies show that if you keep your blood sugar close to normal, you can dramatically reduce your risks of complications. Even if you haven't controlled your blood sugar in the past, it's not too late to start. As soon as you begin managing your sugar level, you slow the progression of the complications you already have, and reduce your chances of developing still more health problems.

Short-term vs. long-term complications

Diabetes can produce two types of complications:

Medical emergencies. Short-term diabetes complications are those that spark medical emergencies requiring immediate attention. This includes low blood sugar, high blood sugar and excessive blood acids.

Development of other diseases. Long-term diabetes complications are those that develop gradually and that may become disabling or life-threatening. They include nerve, kidney, eye, and heart and blood vessel disease.

Low blood sugar (hypoglycemia)

Low blood sugar — a level below 60 milligrams of glucose per deciliter of blood (mg/dL) — is called hypoglycemia (HI-poh-gly-SEE-me-uh). This condition basically results from too much insulin and too little glucose in your blood. Low blood sugar is most common among people taking insulin. Hypoglycemia also can occur in people taking oral medications that enhance the release or action of insulin.

Your blood sugar level can drop for many reasons. Some of the most common include:

- Skipping a meal

- Exercising longer or more strenuously than normal

- Not adjusting your medication to accommodate changes in your blood sugar

What are the signs and symptoms?
Symptoms of hypoglycemia vary, depending on how low your blood sugar level drops.

Early symptoms (blood sugar level of 40 to 55 mg/dL):

- Sweating
- Shakiness
- Visual disturbances

- Weakness
- Hunger
- Dizziness

- Nervousness
- Headache
- Fast heartbeat

- Irritability
- Nausea
- Cold, clammy skin

Later symptoms (blood sugar level below 40 mg/dL):

- Slurred speech
- Drunkenlike behavior

- Drowsiness
- Confusion

Emergency symptoms (blood sugar below 20 mg/dL):

- Convulsions

- Unconsciousness, which can be fatal

Hypoglycemia unawareness

Some people who have had diabetes for several years don't experience early symptoms of low blood sugar, such as shakiness or nervousness. That's because chemical changes from long-standing diabetes may mask the symptoms or keep them from occurring.

With this condition, called hypoglycemia unawareness, you may not realize your blood sugar is low until later symptoms, such as confusion or slurred speech, set in.

What should you do?

As soon as you realize that your blood sugar is low, eat or drink something that will raise your blood sugar level quickly. Good examples include:

- Hard candy, equal to about five Life Savers
- A regular — not diet — soft drink
- Half a cup of fruit juice
- Glucose tablets, nonprescription sugar pills made especially for treating low blood sugar

If after 15 minutes you continue to experience symptoms, repeat the treatment. If they still don't go away, contact your doctor. If you lose consciousness or for some other reason are unable to swallow, the treatment of choice is an injection of glucagon, a fast-acting hormone that stimulates the release of sugar into your blood. You need to teach your close friends and family members how to give you the shot in case of an emergency. Also inform them to call a doctor if the shot doesn't help and you don't regain consciousness.

A glucagon emergency kit includes the medication and a syringe. The shot is easy to administer and is generally given in an arm, buttock, thigh or the abdomen. The medication starts to act in about 5 minutes. If you take insulin, you should have a glucagon kit with or near you at all times. Many people have several kits and keep one in each of their vehicles, at home, at work and in a purse or sports bag.

High blood sugar (diabetic hyperosmolar syndrome)

In this condition your blood sugar reaches such a high level that your blood actually becomes thick and syrupy. Diabetic hyperosmolar syndrome (DHS) may occur with a blood sugar level of 600 mg/dL or higher. Your cells can't absorb this much blood sugar, so the sugar passes from your blood into your urine. This triggers a filtering process that draws tremendous amounts of fluid from your body and produces dehydration.

DHS is most common in people with type 2 diabetes, especially people who don't monitor their blood sugar or who don't know they have diabetes. It can occur in people with diabetes who are taking high-dose steroids or drugs that increase urination. It also may be brought on by an infection, illness, stress or drinking excessive amounts of alcohol.

What are the signs and symptoms?
Symptoms of DHS include:

- Excessive thirst
- Increased urination
- Weakness
- Leg cramps
- Confusion
- Rapid pulse
- Convulsions
- Coma

What should you do?

Check your blood sugar level. If it is 600 mg/dL or higher, see a doctor immediately. Emergency treatment can correct the problem within hours. Doctors may give you intravenous fluids to restore water to your tissues, and short-acting insulin to help your tissue cells absorb glucose. Without prompt treatment, the condition can be fatal.

Increased blood acids (diabetic ketoacidosis)

Diabetic ketoacidosis (DKA) occurs when your muscle cells become so starved for energy that your body takes emergency measures and breaks down fat. As your body transforms the fat into energy, it produces toxic acids known as ketones (KEE-tones).

DKA is most common among people with type 1 diabetes and occurs most often because of insufficient insulin. Perhaps you skipped some of your shots or you didn't raise your insulin dose to adjust for a rise in your blood sugar level. Extreme stress or illness, which can occur in people with either type 1 or type 2 diabetes, also may cause DKA. When you develop an infection, your body produces certain hormones, such as adrenaline, to help fight off the problem. Unfortunately, these hormones also work against insulin. Sometimes the two causes occur together. You get sick or over-stressed, and you forget to take your insulin.

In people who are unaware they have diabetes, a high ketones level can be a warning sign of the disease.

What are the signs and symptoms?

As your level of ketones rises, you may experience any of the following symptoms, many of which can be confused with the flu:

- Deep, rapid breathing
- Sweet, fruity smell on your breath
- Loss of appetite
- Nausea
- Vomiting
- Fever
- Stomach pain

- Weight loss
- Fatigue
- Weakness
- Confusion
- Drowsiness

What should you do?

It's a good idea to check for ketones when you're sick. You should also check for ketones if you're feeling especially stressed or whenever your blood sugar is persistently above 240 mg/dL.

You can buy a ketones test kit at a drugstore or pharmacy and do the test at home. Most kits use chemically treated strips that you dip into your urine. When you have high amounts of ketones in your blood, excess ketones are excreted in your urine. Test strips in the kit change color in accordance with the level of ketones in your urine: low, moderate and high.

If the color on your test strip corresponds with a high ketone level, call your doctor right away. Left untreated, diabetic ketoacidosis can lead to a coma and possibly death. You'll likely need treatment and, perhaps, a hospital stay if:

- You've lost more than 5 percent of your body weight
- You take more than 35 breaths a minute
- You can't control your blood sugar
- You've become confused
- You have more than one bout of nausea and vomiting

Treatment usually involves replenishing lost fluids through intravenous (IV) lines. Insulin, which may be combined with glucose, is injected into an IV so that your body will stop making ketones. Gradually, your blood sugar level is brought back to normal. Adjusting your blood sugar too quickly can produce swelling in your brain. Researchers aren't sure what causes the swelling, but they've observed that the complication is most common in children, especially those with newly diagnosed diabetes.

Nerve damage (neuropathy)

Neuropathy is a common long-term complication of diabetes. You have an intricate network of nerves that runs throughout your body, connecting your brain to muscles, skin and other organs. Through these nerves, your brain senses pain, controls your muscles and performs automatic tasks such as breathing and digestion. High levels of blood sugar can damage these delicate nerves. Excess sugar is thought to weaken the walls of tiny blood vessels (capillaries) that nourish your nerves.

Diabetic neuropathy (noo-ROP-uh-thee) affects 6 out of 10 people with diabetes. Sometimes the results can be painful and disabling. More often symptoms are mild.

What are the signs and symptoms?
There are many kinds of nerve damage. Damage to nerves that control your muscles may leave you with weakened muscles and an unsteady walk. Damage to your autonomic nerves can increase your heart rate and perspiration level. In men, such damage can interfere with their ability to have an erection. Damage to your sensory nerves may leave you unable to detect sensations such as pain, warmth, coolness and texture.

Most commonly, diabetes damages the sensory nerves in your legs, and less often, your arms. You may experience a tingling feeling, numbness, pain or a combination of these sensations. Some people have burning pain that comes and goes. Others have stabbing or aching pain that's worse at night. Still others describe the discomfort as a crawling sensation. The symptoms often begin at the tips of your toes, fingers or both and gradually spread upward. The symptoms may change over time.

Doctors often can detect sensory nerve damage. If, for example, the nerves in a toe are damaged, you won't be able to feel a light pinprick or the vibration of a tuning fork held against the toe. Left untreated, you could lose all sense of feeling in the affected limb, putting you at high risk for injuring your feet without realizing it. Foot care is very important. If you've lost feeling in your feet, and you don't check them each day, you may not realize you have a cut or open wound until serious infection sets in. Nerve damage in a foot that leads to development of an ulcer is the main cause of amputations in people with diabetes. Each year, nearly 60,000 amputations are performed on people with diabetes.

How is it treated?

Good blood sugar control will reduce your symptoms. To help relieve pain, your doctor may prescribe a pain reliever, or an antidepressant or an antiseizure medication that also can reduce pain. Another treatment for nerve-related pain is a nonprescription cream called capsaicin (Zostrix, Trixaicin), which contains hot pepper extract. When you rub the cream on your skin, it helps block pain sensations. Relief usually begins within 2 to 4 weeks after you begin using the cream. To keep the pain from returning, you need to apply the cream daily. Other therapies for pain relief include acupuncture, biofeedback and relaxation techniques.

Because your sensation to hot and cold temperatures may be reduced, it's important that you not burn yourself when bathing or using an electric blanket or heating pad. Also guard against frostbite in cold temperatures.

For more information on impotence resulting from nerve damage, see Chapter 12.

Kidney damage (nephropathy)

Inside your kidneys are millions of tiny blood vessels (capillaries) that filter waste from your blood and dispose of it in your urine. Diabetes can damage this delicate filtering system, often before you notice any symptoms. More than 3 out of 10 people with type 1 diabetes eventually develop kidney disease, called nephropathy (nef-ROP-uh-thee), compared to about 1 in 10 people with type 2 diabetes. Part of the reason for the difference is that people with type 1 diabetes typically develop the disease while at a younger age. The longer you have diabetes, the higher your risk of kidney damage.

What are the signs and symptoms?

In its early stages, kidney disease produces few symptoms. Generally, not until the damage is extensive do symptoms emerge:

- Swelling of the ankles, feet and hands
- Shortness of breath
- High blood pressure

- Confusion or difficulty concentrating
- Poor appetite
- Nausea and vomiting
- Dry, itchy skin
- Fatigue

How is it treated?

Treatment depends on how advanced the disease is. For early disease, keeping your blood sugar level near normal can prevent your condition from getting worse, and possibly improve it. Angiotensin-converting enzyme (ACE) inhibitors — drugs typically used to treat high blood pressure and heart problems — may help slow progression of kidney disease. Another option is to eat a low-protein diet, which seems to reduce the workload of your kidneys. But consult your doctor or dietitian before making changes to your diet.

Treatment for severe damage, known as kidney failure or end-stage renal disease, includes kidney dialysis or a kidney transplant. During kidney dialysis your blood is funneled through a machine that removes waste from it.

Diabetes is the nation's leading cause of kidney failure. For uncertain reasons, kidney failure is escalating among certain races. It's four times more common among blacks than among whites with diabetes. It's also four to six times more common among Hispanics and six times more common among American Indians.

Eye damage (retinopathy)

The back part of your eye, called the retina, is nourished by many tiny vessels. These blood vessels are often among the first to be damaged by high blood sugar.

Nearly everyone with type 1 diabetes and more than 6 out of 10 people with type 2 diabetes develop some form of eye damage by the time they've had diabetes for 20 years. Most people experience only mild vision problems. For others, the effects are more severe, including blindness. Diabetes is the leading cause of blindness in adults in the United States. Each year 12,000 to 24,000 people lose their sight from diabetes.

There are two forms of retinopathy:

Nonproliferative. This form is mild and the most common. Blood vessels in your retina become weak and may swell or develop bulges or fatty deposits. The condition generally doesn't affect your vision unless some of the swollen vessels are in the tiny portion of your retina called the macula, which is responsible for your sharpest vision.

Proliferative. When tiny blood vessels in the retina are damaged, they can bleed or close off. New and fragile blood vessels may form in the retina, and they too may bleed. If this bleeding is heavy or occurs in certain areas of the eye, it can obscure your vision. New blood vessels also can form scar tissue that can push or pull on your retina and distort your vision.

Proliferative retinopathy may require special treatment by an ophthalmologist. Therefore, it's important to catch the disease early so that it can be treated.

What are the signs and symptoms?

Early eye disease often produces few, if any, symptoms. As the damage gradually becomes more severe, the following symptoms may develop:

- "Spiders," "cobwebs" or tiny specks floating in an eye
- A gray shadow in your field of vision
- Blurred vision
- Blurred words while reading
- A dark or empty spot in the center of your vision
- Dark streaks or a red film that blocks vision
- Eye pain
- Flashes of light or rings around objects
- Straight lines that appear distorted
- Vision loss

How is it treated?

Regular eye examinations can identify problems early before permanent damage occurs. Treatment may include a laser procedure to seal weak blood vessels and stop them from leaking. In most cases only one eye is treated at a time. You may need several treatments, which are usually painless. If bleeding into the middle of an eye occurs, you may need a surgical procedure to remove the blood and replace it with a clear fluid that allows light to pass through to the retina.

A displaced or detached retina from buildup of scar tissue generally requires surgery to position the retina in place. Your vision may take several months to improve and in some cases may never fully return.

Heart and blood vessel disease

Diabetes dramatically increases your risk of developing one of many cardiovascular problems, including:

- Chest pain (angina)
- Heart attack
- Stroke
- Narrowing of the arteries to your legs and brain from poor blood circulation (peripheral vascular disease)
- High blood pressure

Diabetes can damage your major arteries, including those that supply blood to your heart and brain. The damage makes it easier for fatty deposits (plaques) to form in the arteries. It also increases pressure in the arteries and reduces blood circulation. Heart disease is the direct cause of more than 77,000 deaths each year among people with diabetes.

What are the signs and symptoms?

Symptoms of heart disease vary. In its early stages, heart disease often produces no symptoms. Later on, warning signs of a heart or blood vessel condition may include:

- Shortness of breath
- Pain in your chest, jaw or arm
- Fatigue and weakness
- Swelling (edema)
- Lightheadedness
- Rapid or irregular heart beats (palpitations)
- Excessive perspiration

People with diabetes are at particular risk for silent (asymptomatic) heart attacks — heart attacks without typical symptoms. Diabetes can damage the nerves that transmit chest pain, which typically accompanies a heart attack. Without pain sensations, people are unaware a heart attack is occurring.

How is it treated?

Many forms of heart disease are treated with medication to prevent symptoms from worsening. If you have accumulation of plaques in your arteries, your doctor may recommend a procedure (angioplasty) to open the arteries. Sometimes surgery is required to bypass clogged arteries leading to your heart.

Other important steps that can help reduce your symptoms and prevent your condition from worsening include eating a healthy diet, getting more exercise, stopping smoking and, if you're overweight, losing weight.

Increased risk of infection

High blood sugar impairs the function of your immune cells to fight off invading germs and bacteria, putting you at higher risk of infection. Your mouth, gums, lungs, skin, feet, bladder and genital area are common infection sites.

High blood sugar also can damage those nerves that would otherwise alert you to a potential infection. An example is your bladder. Damage to nerves that control bladder sensations may fail to alert you that your bladder is full. As a result of constantly being overstretched, your bladder may lose its muscle tone and its ability to empty completely. Bacteria may grow in the remaining urine, causing an infection.

What are the signs and symptoms?
Symptoms of infection vary, depending on its location. A low-grade fever is common with many infections. If the infection is in your gums, you may experience red and bleeding gums. A bladder infection typically causes frequent urination, an urgency to urinate and a burning sensation while urinating. A common symptom of a vaginal infection is itching in the genital area. For a foot wound, redness around the injury site or an accumulation of pus often are warnings of an infection.

How is it treated?
The most common treatment for a bacterial infection is an antibiotic to kill the invading organism. In case of a severe infection, such as a foot injury, your doctor may perform a procedure to clean the injured area and remove infected tissue.

You can reduce your risk of gum disease by brushing and flossing your teeth regularly. You can reduce your risk of a bladder infection by going to the bathroom regularly and making sure to empty your bladder.

Preventing complications

Long-term studies are helping doctors better understand the relationship between blood sugar levels and risk of complications. One of the most important discoveries, confirmed by several studies, is that tight blood sugar control — keeping your blood sugar within a normal or near-normal range — can dramatically reduce your risk of developing many of the complications we've just discussed.

Diabetes Control and Complications Trial (DCCT)
The Diabetes Control and Complications Trial (DCCT), a 10-year study sponsored by the National Institute of Diabetes and Digestive and Kidney Diseases, was conducted from 1983 to 1993. Because

the results were so decisive, its findings were released a year early to allow people with diabetes to take advantage of the new information: Tight blood sugar control can reduce risk of many complications by at least 50 percent.

The study involved 1,441 volunteers with type 1 diabetes. The volunteers were randomly assigned to either conventional treatment or what investigators called intensive treatment.

The conventional group gave themselves one or two injections of insulin daily and had no specific program for testing sugar in their blood or keeping it within a certain range. The intensive therapy group gave themselves three to five insulin injections each day or used continuous-infusion insulin pumps. Their goal was to keep their blood sugar as close to normal as possible — between 80 and 120 mg/dL. This group tested their blood sugar four to seven times a day and adjusted their insulin dosage as needed. They also worked closely with doctors, nurses and dietitians, who helped fine-tune their treatment.

People in the conventional program had an average blood sugar level of 231 mg/dL, compared with 155 mg/dL for the intensive treatment group. And it quickly became apparent that better blood sugar control translated into fewer complications. Fewer people in the intensive therapy group experienced troublesome complications, such as eye or nerve damage, than those receiving conventional treatment.

This study didn't involve people with type 2 diabetes, but researchers felt the findings also would apply to people with type 2 disease.

United Kingdom Prospective Diabetes Study (UKPDS)
The United Kingdom Prospective Diabetes Study (UKPDS) recruited 5,102 people with newly diagnosed type 2 diabetes between 1977 and 1991. Participants were followed for an average of 10 years. The results showed that, overall, people who tried to keep their blood sugar at a normal level had one-fourth fewer complications involving their eyes, kidneys and nerves. Improved blood sugar

and blood pressure control also lead to a reduced risk of heart disease.

Kumamoto study

The Kumamoto study was an 8-year study that included 110 people in Japan with type 2 diabetes who weren't overweight. Members of the group received daily insulin injections, with one group following an intensive insulin therapy program. Compared to people in the conventional program, those who received intensive insulin therapy experienced a delay in the start and progression of eye, kidney and nerve complications.

Questions and answers

If I experience diabetic coma and no one is around to help me, will I eventually come out of it?

A comatose condition can result from dangerously high or low blood sugar. Whether consciousness is regained without assistance depends on many factors, including how high or low your blood sugar level is and how long it has been since you last ate or last received an insulin injection.

If you live alone or are by yourself for much of the day, recruit family members or friends to give you a call if you don't show up for work or to check on you periodically. It may seem like imposing, but these people are often happy to help, and they may even save your life.

If I come across someone who I know has diabetes and he or she appears to be in a coma, how do I know if his or her blood sugar is too high or too low?

There is no way you can tell. The best plan of action is to assume that his or her blood sugar is too low and give the person a glucagon injection. Or if the person is alert enough, get him or her to eat or drink something high in sugar. If the individual doesn't respond within 1 to 2 minutes, call for emergency medical assistance. If the coma is a result of an extremely high blood sugar level, a glucagon injection won't place the person in added danger.

Are people with diabetes who have a heart attack more likely to die from the heart attack than heart attack victims who don't have diabetes?

Yes, risk of death following a heart attack is higher among people with diabetes. One study shows that approximately 6 years following a heart attack, the survival rate is about 50 percent for men and 40 percent for women with diabetes. That compares to survival rates of 70 percent for men and 75 percent for women without diabetes.

People with diabetes are more likely to have high blood pressure and high cholesterol, which increase damage to those arteries that supply oxygen to the heart (coronary arteries), causing a more severe attack. In addition, people with diabetes are less likely to experience typical symptoms of a heart attack, so they may not seek medical attention as quickly.

Can children with diabetes have heart attacks?

Not usually. Though people with type 1 diabetes usually develop the disease as children, they tend not to get heart disease until they reach adulthood. However, diabetes is the leading cause of heart attacks in this country among people below age 30.

How likely am I to already have eye damage by the time I'm diagnosed with diabetes?

About 2 in 10 people with type 2 diabetes have retinopathy when they're first diagnosed. While this initial damage may be minimal and not interfere with normal vision, it increases your susceptibility to more serious eye disease. Because type 1 diabetes develops faster, the percentage of people with retinopathy isn't as high. Most people with type 1 diabetes, however, eventually develop vision problems.

Part 2

Taking Control

Chapter 3

Monitoring your blood sugar

Control. That word comes up again and again, and for good reason. If you have diabetes, controlling your blood sugar (glucose) level is the single most important thing you can do to feel your best and prevent long-term complications.

But how do you achieve control? The cornerstones to controlling diabetes are:

- Monitoring your blood sugar
- Eating a healthy diet
- Staying active
- Maintaining a healthy weight
- Using medications appropriately, when necessary

In this chapter, we focus on the first of these five behaviors. Blood sugar monitoring is essential because to control your blood sugar you must know where it's at. Monitoring is the only way to know whether you're achieving your treatment goals. As one man with diabetes said, "No news is not good news as a diabetic. The more we know about our condition, the better our condition."

If you've just been diagnosed with diabetes, or your treatment has changed, monitoring can seem overwhelming at first. You might feel angry, upset or fearful about having diabetes. You may be anxious about testing — afraid that it will take over your life, that it will be painful or disruptive. These feelings are normal. But as you learn how to measure your blood sugar and understand how regular testing can help you, you'll feel more comfortable doing the procedure and more in control of your disease.

Know your goals

You want your blood sugar to stay within a desirable range — not too high or too low. This range is often referred to as your target range or your blood sugar goal. The normal range for blood sugar before eating is 70 to 110 milligrams of glucose per deciliter of blood (mg/dL). Ideally, that's the level at which you want to keep your blood sugar. But that's not realistic for most people with diabetes. Instead, your focus may be on a range that's near normal.

Your doctor will help you determine your blood sugar goals. Because blood sugar naturally rises following a meal, your goal after meals will be different than before meals. Your goal before bed also may be different than during the day. In determining your goals, your doctor takes into account several factors, including your age, whether you have any diabetes-related complications or other medical conditions, and how good you are at recognizing when your blood sugar is low. Recognizing symptoms of low blood sugar (hypoglycemia) is important because if your blood sugar drops too low, you may lose consciousness or experience a seizure, which can be dangerous.

Among younger adults who don't have complications of diabetes and who can easily recognize symptoms of low blood sugar, a typical target range before meals is 80 to 120 mg/dL. For children the range is often 70 to 120 mg/dL. Approximately $1\frac{1}{2}$ to 2 hours after meals — when blood sugar is often highest — your goal may be to keep your blood sugar level below 180 mg/dL. For older adults who have complications from their disease or people who have trouble recognizing symptoms of low blood sugar, target goals often are higher. Your goal before meals may be 100 to 140 mg/dL, and after meals, less than 200 mg/dL.

When to test

How often you need to test your blood sugar and at what time of day depend on the type of diabetes you have and your treatment plan.

If you take insulin, you should test your blood sugar frequently, at least twice a day and preferably three or four times a day. Some people measure their blood sugar five or six times a day. Testing is normally done before meals and at bedtime — in other words, when you haven't eaten for 4 or more hours. It's best to test your blood sugar just before your insulin injection. In some circumstances you may want to test after a meal as well.

Many people who use a rapid-acting insulin check their blood sugar $1\frac{1}{2}$ to 2 hours after eating to see if the insulin is working properly and keeping their blood sugar within their goal. A change in your regular routine may be another reason to test your blood sugar, especially if you have type 1 diabetes. This may include exercising more than normal, eating less than usual or traveling. Special circumstances, including pregnancy or illness, also may warrant increased testing.

For people with type 2 diabetes who don't use insulin, the frequency of testing is more varied. You want to test your blood sugar as often as is necessary to keep it in good control. For some people this may mean daily testing, while for others it might be twice a week. In general, people who are able to control their blood sugar with diet and exercise, and without use of medication, don't need to test their blood sugar as often.

Your doctor or a diabetes educator can help you determine a monitoring schedule that's right for you.

Tools you need

Testing your blood sugar is a quick and easy process that generally takes less than 2 minutes. Here's what you need:

A lancet. A lancet is a small needle that pricks the skin on your finger so that you can draw a drop of blood. Spring-loaded lancets are generally less painful.

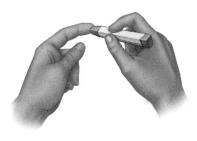

Test strips. Test strips are chemically treated strips onto which you place blood from your finger. Most blood glucose monitors sold today require that you insert the strip into the monitor first, before drawing blood from your finger. With older models the strip is inserted after blood is applied to it.

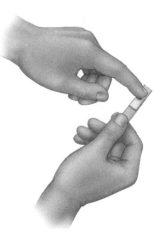

Blood glucose monitor. A blood glucose monitor, also called a blood glucose meter, is a small, computerized devise that measures and displays your blood sugar level.

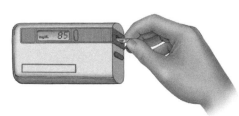

Performing the test

Before pricking your finger, wash your hands with soap and warm water. Dry them well. Don't use alcohol to clean your finger because it can alter the test results. Remove a test strip from the container and replace the cap immediately to prevent damage to the strips. With a lancet, stick the side of your finger, not the tip, so that you won't have sore spots on the part of your finger you use the most. (Your fingertips also have the most nerve endings.) Rotate the sites where you stick your fingers. When you have a drop of blood, apply it to the test strip and wait for a reading. Within a few seconds the meter displays your blood sugar level on a screen.

Getting a good reading

Blood glucose monitors are generally accurate and precise. Human error rather than a nonfunctioning machine is more likely to produce an inaccurate reading. To ensure accurate results, follow each step carefully. Problems that can lead to an inaccurate reading include:

- Not enough blood applied to the test strip
- More blood added to the test strip after the first drop was applied
- Alcohol, dirt or other substances on your finger
- Damaged or outdated test strips

Choosing the right monitor

Blood glucose monitors come in many forms with a variety of features. So how do you know which device is right for you? Your diabetes educator or doctor may recommend a specific monitor or help you select one. Also keep in mind that some health plans require their participants to use a particular monitor.

When choosing a monitor, consider these factors:

Cost. Most insurance plans, as well as Medicare, cover the cost of a blood glucose monitor and test strips. But some plans limit the total number of test strips allowed. Monitors range in price from $30 to $150 or more. The same monitor can differ in price by as much as $50, so shop around before you buy.

The test strips are the most expensive part of monitoring. They generally cost $30 to $40 for a container of 50. Strips that are individually packaged tend to cost more, but you might not use all the strips in a container before the expiration date, or within 90 days of opening the container. Figure out which type of strip is most cost-effective for you.

Ease of use and maintenance. Some monitors are easier to use than others. Are the monitor and strips comfortable to hold? Can you easily see the numbers on the screen? How easy is it to get blood onto the strips? Find out how the monitor is calibrated, that is, how it is set for the test strips you'll use. How often will you have to recalibrate the monitor? How often do you have to change the batteries?

Special features. Many monitors are designed to meet specific needs. Some monitors are larger, with strips that are easier to handle. Some strips siphon blood from your fingertip rather than requiring you to place a drop of blood on them. For kids there are colorful monitors that give a quicker reading. People with impaired vision can buy a monitor with a large screen or a talking monitor.

Also consider how the monitor stores and retrieves information. Some can track all the information you would normally write in a log, such as the time and date of a test, the result and trends over time. You can even download this information into a computer to chart your diabetes management.

- A damaged meter
- A dirty meter, especially the test window
- A meter that's not at room temperature
- A meter not coded for the test strips

An easy way to check your meter and your testing skill is to bring your meter with you when you have a doctor's appointment.

Are you getting quality results?

To do a quality control test, follow your normal blood-testing procedure, but use a liquid control solution instead of blood. These solutions are available at most drugstores and pharmacies and come in three ranges: high, normal or low. Ask your diabetes educator which solution to use.

Acceptable values for the control test are listed in the insert that comes with the control solution or with the test strips. If the results of your control test don't fall within the acceptable range, do the following:

Check the strips. Throw out damaged or out-of-date strips.

Check the control solution. Check the expiration date and use fresh solution, if necessary.

Check the meter. Make sure the strip guide and the test window are clean. Follow the manufacturer's instructions for cleaning. Replace batteries if they're weak.

Check the calibration (measurement scale) of the meter. Some meters are calibrated in the factory and have a check strip or paddle that can be inserted to verify the calibration. Others are calibrated to each container of strips. Make sure you're using strips that have been calibrated for your meter. If indicated, be sure the code number in the meter matches the code number on the strip container.

After you've corrected potential problems, repeat the control test. If the results are still unacceptable, talk to your diabetes educator or call the meter manufacturer for assistance.

If possible do a quality control test once a week. It's also a good idea to do the test when you start a new container of test strips or you calibrate the meter or charge the batteries.

Your doctor, nurse or diabetes educator will have you check your blood sugar at the same time blood is drawn for laboratory tests. That way you can compare the reading you get with the lab results. Your meter results shouldn't be off by more than 15 percent.

It's also a good idea to periodically perform a quality control test of your equipment and technique. (See "Are you getting quality results?")

Recording your results

More than just providing an immediate measurement of your blood sugar, monitoring can help you assess your progress in managing your diabetes. Each time you perform a blood test, log your results. The information you write down helps you see how food, physical activity, medication and other factors affect your blood sugar. As patterns emerge you begin to understand how your daily activities affect your blood sugar level. This puts you in a better position to manage your diabetes day by day and even hour by hour.

Your life is not the same from one day to the next. Some days you exercise more or eat less. Maybe you're sick or you're having trouble at work or home. These changes affect your blood sugar level. By keeping an accurate record of day-to-day events and your blood sugar levels, you'll find problem areas and will be better able to maintain good control.

With the information you gain, you can anticipate problems before they occur. You can plan ahead for changes in your routine that you know will affect your blood sugar, such as traveling, eating out or working overtime.

Your diabetes educator or doctor may have given you a record book for recording your test results. If not, you can use any type of notebook. You also can keep your results on computer. Many software programs are available for recording and tracking blood sugar levels. Every time you check your blood sugar, write down:

- The date and time
- The test result
- The type and dosage of medication you're taking

You also may want to include other information that can help explain a deviation from your normal blood sugar level:

- A change in your diet, such as having a birthday dinner, eating at a restaurant or eating more than usual
- A change in your exercise or activity level
- Unusual excitement or stress
- An illness
- An insulin reaction

Sample record: Intensive insulin therapy

Day and date	Insulin type	Insulin dosage (number of units taken)					Blood glucose and urine ketone test results										Comments (changes in diet and activity, weight, insulin reactions, illness, etc.)
		Breakfast	Noon meal	Evening meal	Bedtime snack			Breakfast Before	After	Breakfast Before	After	Breakfast Before	After	Bedtime	During night		
Sunday						Time											
						BG											
	Supp.					UK											
Monday						Time											
						BG											
	Supp.					UK											
Tuesday						Time											
						BG											
	Supp.					UK											
Wednesday						Time											
						BG											
	Supp.					UK											
Thursday						Time											
						BG											
	Supp.					UK											
Friday						Time											
						BG											
	Supp.					UK											
Saturday						Time											
						BG											
	Supp.					UK											

Sample record: Standard drug therapy

Date	Medication dose	Blood glucose test results				Comments (changes in diet and activity, weight, insulin reactions, illness, urine ketones, etc.)
		Before breakfast	Before noon meal	Before evening meal	Before bedtime meal	

Bring your record book with you when you see your doctor, diabetes educator or dietitian. He or she can help you interpret the results. Based on the information you keep, your doctor can help you make changes in your medication and lifestyle. The more complete your records are, the more useful they'll be.

Magic numbers

When you're testing and recording your blood sugar frequently, it's easy to get caught up in a numbers game. The right numbers equal success, while the wrong numbers represent failure. You may end up feeling upset, confused, angry, frustrated or discouraged about your blood sugar results. It's easy to judge yourself on your numbers. Good numbers, good person — bad numbers, bad person.

It's also easy to become obsessive about testing and test results. If you're already a perfectionist or on the obsessive side, you can go overboard with all the numbers and record keeping involved in monitoring your blood sugar.

There's nothing magical about these numbers. They're not a judgment of you as a person. They're a tool to help you track how well your treatment plan is working. Your results can indicate if you need to make changes in your treatment. No matter how well you're doing with your plan or how hard you try, your blood sugar readings won't be perfect every time. Sometimes "bad" readings happen for no apparent reason.

Factors that affect blood sugar

The amount of sugar in your blood continuously varies. That's because many factors affect how your body metabolizes food into sugar and how it uses this sugar. Self-monitoring helps you learn what makes your blood sugar level rise and fall so that you can make adjustments in your treatment. It also can help you understand why your blood sugar level may be different from day to day or hour to hour.

Food

Food raises your blood sugar level. One to 2 hours after a meal, your blood sugar is at its highest level, then it starts to fall. What you eat, how much you eat and at what time you eat all affect your blood sugar level.

Strive for consistency from day to day in the time you eat and the amount of food you eat. By controlling when and how much you eat, you control the times your blood sugar is higher, such as after meals. You also control how high your blood sugar rises. If you eat too much, your blood sugar will be higher than usual. Too little food may result in lower than usual blood sugar. If you take insulin, this could put you at risk of hypoglycemia (see page 22).

It's also important to understand that different foods have a different effect on your blood sugar. Food is made up of carbohydrates, protein and fat. All three increase blood sugar, but carbohydrates have the most noticeable effect. Even within the carbohydrates group, different types have varying affects on blood sugar.

Your liver

Sugar is stored in your liver in a form called glycogen. Your liver also makes new sugar from other substances, such as protein and fat. When your blood sugar level falls, your liver breaks down glycogen and releases it into your bloodstream. This generally happens when you haven't eaten for a while. The continuous process of storing and releasing sugar causes natural fluctuations in your blood sugar level.

Exercise and activity

Typically, exercise and physical activity lower your blood sugar level. With help from insulin, exercise promotes the transfer of sugar from your blood to your cells, where the sugar is used for energy. The more you exercise, the more sugar you use and the faster it's transported to the cells, thereby lowering the amount of sugar in your blood. Exercise also reduces insulin resistance, making your cells more accepting of insulin.

Exercise can lower your blood sugar for several hours, and sometimes excessively. Some people find that strenuous activity reduces their blood sugar for 1 or 2 days. That's why it's always prudent to be prepared for a low blood sugar reaction during and following exercise.

Although fairly uncommon, sometimes exercise has the opposite effect — it raises your blood sugar. This usually happens if your blood sugar is very high to begin with — typically more than 300 mg/dL. When blood sugar is this high, exercise causes your body to release or produce extra sugar, and not enough insulin is available to use it. If you take insulin, an increase in blood sugar also may happen if your insulin level is very low when you start exercising. Until you know how your body responds to exercise, you should test your blood sugar before and after exercising and again several hours later.

Physical activity such as housework, gardening or being on your feet all day also affects your blood sugar. Generally, the more active you are, the lower your blood sugar. Similar to exercise, physical activity promotes energy expenditure. You'll want to monitor your blood sugar level and make adjustments in your medications to match your activity level, especially if you deviate from your normal routine.

Medications

Insulin and oral diabetes medications lower your blood sugar level. The time of day you take your medication and how much you take affect how much your blood sugar level drops. If your medication is causing your blood sugar to drop too much, or not enough, your doctor may need to make adjustments to your dosage.

Medications taken for other conditions also can affect blood sugar. Whenever you're prescribed a new medication for a health condition, make sure to let your doctor know that you have diabetes and ask if the medication may alter your blood sugar level.

You may still need to take a medication that affects your blood sugar because of its benefits in treating another health condition. But by being aware of its effects and following simple precautions, such as increased blood sugar monitoring, you can keep it from causing significant changes in your blood sugar levels. If the drug does make it more difficult for you to control your blood sugar, contact your doctor.

Illness

The physical stress of a cold, influenza or other illness, especially a bacterial infection, causes your body to produce hormones that increase blood sugar. Trauma or a major illness like a heart attack also can increase blood sugar. The additional sugar helps to promote healing. But in people with diabetes, more sugar can be a problem. When you're sick it's important to monitor your blood sugar frequently.

Alcohol

Alcohol prevents your liver from releasing sugar and can increase the risk of your blood sugar falling too low. If you take insulin or oral diabetes medications, you risk experiencing low blood sugar (hypoglycemia) when you drink alcohol — even as little as 2 ounces (about two drinks). If you choose to drink alcohol, drink only in moderation. To prevent your blood sugar from dropping too low, never drink on an empty stomach or if your blood sugar is already low.

Less commonly, alcohol can do the opposite — cause your blood sugar to rise. The increase is due to the high number of calories in alcohol. Monitor your blood sugar before and after consuming alcohol to see how your body responds to its use.

When test results signal a problem

A pattern to watch out for is blood sugar readings that are persistently above or below your goals. This might indicate that your medication needs to be adjusted or, if you're not taking medication, that improving your diet and getting more exercise aren't enough to control your blood sugar. Persistent high or low blood sugar readings also may signal an emerging complication of diabetes.

Having high or low blood sugar once in a while — especially if you can pinpoint the reason — isn't cause for alarm. However, frequent, unexplained high or low blood sugar readings need medical attention.

Call your doctor if:

- Your blood sugar is persistently higher than 300 mg/dL.
- Your blood sugar readings are persistently above or below your goals.
- Your blood sugar is greater than 250 mg/dL for more than 24 hours during an illness.
- You have repeated low blood sugars.

New technologies

Sticking yourself with a lancet several times a day is no one's idea of a good time. It can be inconvenient and painful. That's one reason many people don't test their blood sugar as often as they should. Fortunately, lancing devices and blood glucose monitors are always improving. Less invasive and faster devices are now on the market or in development.

Specialized lancing devices

Some lancets can be set for different prick depths to accommodate differences in skin thickness. These devices generally cost between $10 and $30. You also can purchase a needle-free lancing device that uses a laser beam to break the skin on your finger. However, the product costs approximately $1,000 and it may still cause some discomfort.

New glucose monitors

Advances in monitoring include:

All-in-one lancet and monitor. An all-in-one lancet and monitor is a device that uses a drop of blood drawn from an arm or thigh. Because fewer nerve endings are in these areas, the stick should be less painful. The device also requires less blood. All-in-one lancets and monitors are priced around $60.

Wristwatch monitor. A wristwatch monitor is worn around a wrist. It detects blood sugar levels through your skin. Readings are taken every 20 minutes, using a low-level electrical current to extract fluid beneath your skin and draw it to a sensor pad on the back of the watch. An alarm sounds if your blood sugar level rises too high or drops too low. Finger-prick tests are still required at least every 12 hours to calibrate the monitor. The approximate cost is $300.

Other technologies. One type of monitoring system being developed involves wearing a patch on your arm for several minutes. The patch draws glucose from fluid in your skin, and results are read with a portable meter.

Also in the works is a continuous glucose monitor that's implanted under the skin in your lower chest or upper abdomen.

Overcoming barriers to testing

Despite its advantages, many people with diabetes don't test their blood sugar as often as they should — or at all. There are many reasons why:

Cost. Many diabetes supply companies offer low- or no-cost supplies. In addition, many diabetes drug companies have patient assistance programs. If cost is a factor for you, talk with your doctor or diabetes educator. He or she might know of a local or nationwide program that can help defray your expenses.

Limited access to quality care. Many towns, cities and counties have services specifically for people who have trouble accessing health care. If getting to a medical center is a problem, you might check with your county or state health department about outreach health care services.

Lack of information and misperceptions. Some people are simply unaware of the benefits of blood sugar monitoring and believe there is nothing they can do to improve their disease. One of the best weapons in managing diabetes is education. Learn as much as you can about your disease.

Fear. If you fear the discomfort of pricking your finger, keep in mind that newer lancets are less painful. You also shouldn't fear checking your blood sugar in public. With the increase in the number of people with diabetes, blood sugar monitoring has become a more acceptable practice. Millions of people do it every day.

Lifestyle issues. Many people with diabetes have found ways to build monitoring into their daily routine, even with hectic or unconventional work schedules. Your doctor or diabetes educator can help you adjust your monitoring to your particular schedule.

Privacy issues. Testing is quick and monitors are portable. If privacy is important to you, you should be able to find a private place, such as a bathroom, to do your tests.

The sensor measures your glucose level and transmits the information to a pagerlike device worn outside your body.

Yet another technology in development uses near-infrared light beams to determine your blood sugar level. The light shines through tissue packed with small blood vessels, such as an earlobe or fingertip, and extrapolates blood sugar data based on the concentration of sugar in the tissue.

Questions and answers

Should I be testing sugar in my urine? Is that done any more?
In the past, the only practical way for people with diabetes to monitor their blood sugar was by testing sugar in their urine. But urine glucose tests aren't as accurate as blood glucose tests. They provide only a rough estimate of your blood sugar level and can't detect levels below 180 mg/dL. Urine glucose testing is recommended only if blood testing isn't an option.

One type of urine test that is recommended for people with diabetes is a urine ketone test. Ketones are acids that are formed when your body breaks down fat for energy, due to insufficient insulin. When ketones build up in your blood, they can spill over into your urine — an indication that your diabetes may be out of control. For more on ketones, see page 25.

Does stress affect blood sugar?
Stress can affect blood sugar in two ways. When you're under a lot of stress, it's easy to abandon your usual routine. You may exercise less, eat less healthy foods and not test your blood sugar as often. As a result stress indirectly causes your blood sugar to rise.

Occasionally, stress can have a direct effect on your blood sugar level. Physical and psychological stress may cause your body to produce hormones that prevent insulin from working properly, increasing blood sugar levels. This tends to be more common in people with type 2 diabetes. The effect of stress on people with type 1 diabetes is more mixed. Sometimes blood sugar goes down under stress.

To find out how you react to stress, log your stress level on a scale of 1 to 10 every time you log your blood sugar level. After a couple of weeks, look for a pattern. Do high blood sugar levels often occur with high stress levels and low blood sugars with low stress? If so, stress may be affecting your blood sugar control.

Can heat affect my blood sugar level?

Heat doesn't have a direct affect on your blood sugar, but it might lead you to change your daily routine. On hot days, for example, you may eat less than usual or exert yourself more. These changes could lower your blood sugar. Whenever your daily routine changes, test your blood sugar more often.

Sunburn also can affect blood sugar control. A severe sunburn is stressful to the body, and like other physical stresses, it can raise your blood sugar. Use a good sunscreen and wear sunglasses and a hat when you're out in the sun.

What's the difference between whole blood glucose levels and plasma blood glucose levels?

Home blood glucose monitors use whole blood to measure blood sugar. The equipment used in laboratories uses only the plasma portion of your blood. The red blood cells are removed before glucose is measured. Because of this difference, results from laboratories and home monitors aren't exactly the same.

Plasma test results are 10 percent to 15 percent higher than whole blood test results, and they tend to be more accurate. Even though they use whole blood for the test, many home monitors are calibrated to give a plasma test result.

There's no need to worry about the difference between the two as long as your test strips are calibrated correctly to your monitor. Your home monitor's results are considered accurate if they fall within 15 percent of the lab test result.

Do I need to adjust my monitoring routine when I'm traveling?

You can still get out and see the world if you have diabetes. It just takes a little more planning. When you travel bring at least twice the medication and testing supplies as you think you'll need. Because stress, time changes and changes in your eating and sleeping schedule can affect your blood glucose level, it's a good idea to test it more frequently than normal. If you're flying, especially for a long period, test your blood sugar level as soon as possible after landing. Jet lag can make you tired or fatigued, making it more difficult to tell if you have low or high blood sugar.

Chapter 4

Developing a healthy eating plan

The words *healthy eating* often produce a twinge of fear. Many people think, "Oh no, I'll never get to eat anything I like again!" This is a common response when people first hear they have diabetes. That's because people associate the disease with bland, tasteless food.

There's no need to panic. You can still eat foods you enjoy. You may, however, have to limit their amount or change how you prepare them or when you eat them. Healthy eating is not about deprivation or denial. It means enjoying great nutrition as well as great taste. Because your body is a complex machine, it needs a variety of foods to achieve a balanced mix of energy. For people with diabetes, a healthy diet is key to a healthy life.

There is no 'diabetes diet'

Contrary to popular myth, having diabetes doesn't mean that you have to start eating specialized foods or follow a highly detailed and boring diet plan. For most people, having diabetes simply translates into variety and moderation — eating more of certain foods, such as fruits, vegetables and grains that are high in nutrients and low in fat and calories, and less of others, such as animal products and sweets. It's the same eating plan that all Americans should follow.

Depending on your blood sugar (glucose) level, whether you need to lose weight and whether you have other health problems, you may need to tailor your diet somewhat to meet your personal needs. But even though the details may differ, the basics remain the same. Each day you want to eat a variety of foods to achieve the right balance of three key nutrients:

- Carbohydrates
- Protein
- Fats

Carbohydrates: The foundation

Carbohydrates are your body's main energy source. Your brain, for example, uses carbohydrates as its primary source of fuel. At the base of all carbohydrates are sugar components. Depending on the number of components and how they're linked together, a carbohydrate is classified as a simple carbohydrate (sugar) or a complex carbohydrate (starch). During digestion, complex carbohydrates are broken down into simple sugars. Simple sugars are found in sweets, milk, fruit and some vegetables. Complex carbohydrates are found in grain products and certain vegetables.

To help with meal planning, the American Diabetes Association divides carbohydrates into four groups:

Starches. Starches are complex carbohydrates and include bread, cereal, rice, pasta, beans and certain vegetables, such as corn, potatoes and squash.

Fruits. Every form of fruit, from the familiar apples, bananas and oranges to the exotic kumquats, persimmons and prickly pears, contain simple sugars.

Milk products. Milk and milk products contain simple sugars.

Vegetables. This group includes all nonstarchy vegetables, such as lettuce, asparagus and zucchini.

About half your daily calories should come from carbohydrates. Depending on your calorie needs, that might include:

- Six or more servings of starches
- Two to four servings of fruit
- Two to three servings of milk products
- Three to five servings of vegetables

Combining your carbs

It's best to eat a mixture of complex and simple carbohydrates. The advantage of complex carbohydrates is that it takes your body longer to break them down into sugar. Therefore sugar enters your bloodstream at a more prolonged rate. With some simple carbohydrates, sugar may enter your bloodstream quickly.

You also want to include in your carbohydrate mix those that are high in fiber. The more fiber the food contains, the more slowly it's digested and the more slowly your blood sugar level rises. A recent study underscores the benefits of fiber. It suggests that a diet high in fiber may lower blood sugar and blood cholesterol levels in people with type 2 diabetes. Study participants spent 6 weeks on a daily diet containing 25 grams (g) of fiber — the recommended amount for all Americans — followed by another 6 weeks on an experimental diet containing 50 g of fiber daily. Participants ate a variety of fiber-rich fruits, vegetables and grains, including cantaloupe, oranges, raisins, lima beans, sweet potatoes, zucchini and oatmeal. Researchers found that the experimental diet reduced blood sugar levels by about 10 percent, similar to the effects of some medications.

The most important thing about carbohydrates, however, is not so much what type you eat but how much. If you eat more carbohydrates than usual, you may not have enough available insulin to transport the excess sugar to your cells, causing an increase in your blood sugar level. One way you can help control your blood sugar is by eating the same amount of carbohydrates, spaced apart throughout the day.

The scoop on sugar

For decades, people with diabetes were told to avoid sugar. And that's still a common misconception when people first learn they have diabetes — that they'll have to give up sweets for good. But things have changed. Here's why.

For years, medical professionals assumed that honey, candy and other sweets would raise your blood sugar faster and higher than fruits, vegetables or foods containing complex carbohydrates. So people with diabetes were told to avoid sugar. But many studies

Sugar by any other name tastes as sweet

Sugar travels under many guises, depending on how it's formed and how it's produced. Basic table sugars include molasses, beet sugar, cane sugar, white sugar, brown sugar, confectioners' sugar, powdered sugar, raw sugar, turbinado and maple syrup. Regular sugar is also called sucrose. Other kinds of sugars include glucose (dextrose), fructose, lactose, maltose and the sugar alcohols sorbitol, xylitol and mannitol.

When you're shopping, look for these names on product labels. A sweet food may not simply state "sugar" on the label.

have shown this isn't true. All carbohydrates affect blood glucose in about the same way, and sweets don't produce an exaggerated rise in blood sugar, provided they're eaten with your meal and counted as a carbohydrate source.

It's still best to eat sugar in moderation. Eaten in larger amounts, sugar may have a more noticeable effect on your blood sugar. Sweet foods, such as candy, cookies or soda pop, also have little nutritional value. You receive empty calories void of the nutrients your body needs to function. In addition, those extra calories can lead to weight gain.

After eating a sugary food, test your blood sugar and observe its effect, which may differ with different types of sweets. Alternatives to sugar are sugar-free products that contain artificial sweeteners. But keep in mind that some of these "sugar-free" foods may still be high in carbohydrates and calories.

Protein: The power

Your body uses protein for growth, maintenance and energy. Foods high in protein include meat, poultry, eggs, cheese, fish, legumes and peanut butter. If you eat more protein than you need — which many people do — your body stores the extra calories from protein as fat.

For most people, a healthy diet includes 10 percent to 20 percent of their daily calories from protein, or about two to three protein servings. When planning your meals, select proteins that are lower in fat, such as plant products, fish, poultry without skin, lean meats and low-fat or fat-free cheese. Limit or avoid fatty meats, eggs and high-fat cheeses.

Plant sources of protein include legumes — beans, dried peas and lentils — and products made from soy — miso, seitan, tempeh and tofu. In addition to being high in protein, these foods also are low in fat and cholesterol. Never heard of some of these foods? Consider this an opportunity to try something new. Tempeh, for

Special diets

If you have another health condition in addition to diabetes, such as high blood pressure or kidney disease, your doctor may recommend that you follow a diet that helps that condition.

Sodium-controlled diet

Limiting the amount of sodium you eat prevents excessive sodium accumulation in your body. This helps reduce blood pressure and the tendency to retain fluids. Limiting sodium also may help your heart work more effectively.

Salt (sodium chloride) and sodium preservatives added to many processed foods make up the majority of sodium people consume. A sodium-controlled diet avoids or limits foods that are especially high in salt, such as salted snacks, frozen convenience foods, pickles, bacon and soy sauce.

Protein- and potassium-controlled diet

When you have kidney disease, your kidneys have problems performing their normal functions, including regulating the amount of sodium, potassium, calcium and phosphorus in your body, and removing waste products that are produced when protein is broken down.

If your kidneys aren't functioning properly, these minerals and protein by-products can build up in your blood and tissues, and you may need to tailor your diet to limit their consumption. A dietitian can help you learn what foods to eat and which to avoid.

example, has a nutty flavor and meatlike texture. Sounds strange, perhaps, but it makes a great sandwich.

Fats: The calorie heavyweights

Fats are the most concentrated source of food energy, providing lots of calories but little nutritional value. Fats are found in meat, poultry, fish, cheese, butter, margarine, oils, salad dressing, whole milk and many desserts and snack foods. Your body needs some fat to function. It's when you eat too much fat that problems can occur.

Not all fats are created equal. Fats may be saturated, polyunsaturated, monosaturated or a mixture of these. Polyunsaturated and monounsaturated fats, found in seafood, olive oil, canola oil, nuts and avocados, are healthier than saturated fats, found in animal products, such as meat, cream and butter. Still, all fats are very high in calories, no matter what the type.

Cutting down on fat

Limiting the amount of fat you eat will help control blood sugar and blood fats. Follow these tips:

- Read the labels on processed foods and check for fat types and amounts.
- Choose fat-free or low-fat products.
- Use canola or olive oil in small amounts for cooking and salads.
- Avoid fried foods. Instead, bake, steam, grill, broil or roast meat and vegetables. Marinate meats and use herbs and spices to give them flavor.
- Buy lean cuts of meat and trim off the excess fat. Remove the skin from poultry before cooking.
- Season vegetables with lemon, lime or herbs rather than butter or oil.
- Replace shortening in baked goods with applesauce or prune purée.

All Americans, including people with diabetes, should limit total fat consumption to 30 percent or less of their daily calories and saturated fat to no more than 10 percent of their daily calories. Saturated fat raises blood cholesterol, and high blood cholesterol is a risk factor for heart disease.

Planning your meals

A meal plan is simply a guide for eating. It helps you choose the right kinds and amount of foods. The first step in meal planning is to establish a routine of eating meals and snacks at regular times every day. Some people can keep their blood sugar in good control simply by eating three regular meals a day and avoiding excessive sweets. Others need to follow a more deliberate plan, eating only the recommended number of servings from each food group every day, based on their individual calorie needs.

If you haven't been following any particular eating plan and want to develop a more healthy one, start by keeping a log of everything you eat. You may be eating more than you realize, or fewer fruits and vegetables than you'd like. After you've assessed your eating patterns, you and your dietitian can develop a meal plan based on your food preferences and recommended daily calories.

When you're first diagnosed with diabetes, we advise that you talk with your doctor or a dietitian about meal planning. He or she can provide you with a variety of tools to help you prepare healthy, tasty meals. Depending on your progress, you may want to meet with a dietitian on a regular basis. You might not achieve the ideal eating plan right away, but what counts is that you continue to work toward your goal, making gradual improvements.

Working with a dietitian

Understanding what foods to eat, how much to eat and how your food choices affect your blood sugar level can be a complex task. A registered dietitian can help you make sense of all this information and put together a meal plan that's easy for you to follow and that fits your health goals, food tastes, family or cultural traditions and lifestyle.

When you first meet with a dietitian, he or she will ask you questions about your weight and your eating habits — what you like to eat, how much you eat, when and what time of day. The dietitian will then sit down with you and work out a meal plan, taking into account your diabetes treatment goals, your eating habits, work schedule, activity level, calorie needs, whether you're trying to lose weight, any special health considerations and what medications you take.

Meal planning is often a negotiation process. Your dietitian will look at what you're doing now and what your goal is. Together you'll figure out what is practical and achievable for you. For example, say you eat breakfast at a local restaurant with your buddies every Tuesday morning. You usually have two eggs, three pancakes, two pieces of bacon and coffee. Your dietitian understands that this breakfast is an important part of your social life, so he or she isn't going to ask you to give it up. But your dietitian will help you look at other food choices that may fit better into your overall plan. Maybe you'll decide you can get by with one egg, one piece of bacon, two pieces of toast and coffee. A dietitian can walk you through each meal in this way.

Consistency is key

Every day try to eat:

- At the same time

- About the same amount of food

- The same proportion of carbohydrates, protein and fats

This will help keep your blood sugar at a consistent level. It's more difficult to control your blood sugar if you eat a big lunch one day and a small one the next. Also, the more food you eat at one time, the higher your blood sugar will rise. Eating at regularly spaced intervals — meals spaced 4 to 5 hours apart — reduces large variations in blood sugar and also allows for adequate digestion and metabolism of food. If you take insulin, consistent meal times also allow you to eat when you have the greatest insulin action.

Portion police

With the trend toward supersizing, megabuffets and huge portions in restaurants, many people have an inaccurate idea of what a regular portion is. Pay close attention to portion sizes. Don't just estimate.

At first, the serving sizes may seem very small. Three cups of popped popcorn would hardly make a dent in the large bucket you're used to getting at the movies. A 2- to 3-ounce serving of meat may be less than the 8-ounce steak you're used to eating. With time though, you'll find that smaller servings allow you to enjoy a greater variety of foods.

Sizing up a serving

Here are some examples of what counts as one serving:

Food	Serving examples
Starches/grains	1 slice whole-wheat bread
	½ bagel or English muffin
	½ cup cooked cereal, rice or pasta
	¾ cup ready-to-eat cereal
	1 medium potato
Fruits/vegetables	½ cup 100 percent fruit juice
	1 small apple or banana
	1 cup raw, leafy green vegetables
	½ cup cooked vegetables
Milk products	1 cup low-fat or fat-free milk
	1 cup low-fat or fat-free yogurt
Meat/meat substitutes	2 oz. cooked, skinless poultry, seafood or lean meat
	¼ cup low-fat cottage cheese
	½ cup cooked beans, dried peas or lentils

Exchange lists

If you're following a meal plan that you developed with your dietitian, you may be using a booklet that lists foods by food group and serving size, called an exchange list. The exchange system is one tool to help you manage your diet. Not everyone with diabetes needs to use an exchange list, but many people with both type 1 and type 2 diabetes find it helpful.

In the exchange system, foods are grouped into starches, vegetables, fruits, meats, milk products and fats. The foods also are portioned to measure and control calories, carbohydrates and other nutrients. An exchange is basically one portion of a food type. One starch exchange, for instance, might be one small baked potato. You can exchange or trade foods within a group because they're similar in nutrient content and the manner in which they affect your blood sugar.

A dietitian can help you use an exchange list to figure out your daily meal plan. He or she will recommend a certain number of servings from each food group based on your individual needs. Say your goal is 1,400 calories a day. Your dietitian may recommend that you have six or seven starch exchanges (servings), three fruit exchanges, two milk exchanges, six meat or meat substitute exchanges and three to five vegetable exchanges.

Calculating exchanges for recipes

Your meal plan looks great, but there's one small problem: Where do your favorite recipes fit in? They're not on the food lists.

By following the steps below, you can figure out the exchange values for many of your favorite recipes and the number of exchanges each serving of a recipe provides.

1. List all the ingredients in a recipe and their amounts.
2. For each ingredient, write down the number of exchanges it provides. You'll probably have to consult a list of exchange values of commonly used ingredients. You can find this in many diabetic cookbooks or ask your dietitian for one.
3. Total each exchange group.
4. Divide the total number of exchanges for each group by the number of servings in the recipe and round off to the nearest $1/2$ exchange (round up for amounts greater than $1/2$ exchange).

Carb counting

Some people with diabetes — especially those taking multiple injections of insulin or using an insulin pump — calculate their meal-related insulin doses based on the carbohydrate content of the meal. The amount of protein and fat in the meal generally isn't taken into consideration. During each meal and at snack time, they calculate the amount of carbohydrates in the meal or snack and adjust their insulin dose to the carbohydrate count. This helps keep their blood sugar at an optimal level throughout the day.

Because most people with type 1 diabetes are at or below their ideal body weight, they often don't need to be as concerned about the number of calories they eat. However, too many or too few calories can influence blood sugar. Carbohydrate counting is less effective for people with type 2 diabetes because many are overweight and calories and fat are a concern. To lose weight or maintain a healthy weight, you need to consider the total number of calories you eat, not just the carbohydrate calories.

Carbohydrate counting isn't an excuse to go overboard on foods that are low in carbohydrates or don't contain any carbohydrates, such as meat and fats. Remember that too many calories and too much fat and cholesterol over the long term can put you at increased risk of weight gain, heart disease and stroke.

Keeping motivated

It's easy to arm yourself with meal plans, exchange lists and food logs. But it's not always so easy to follow your meal plan day after day. Sticking to a healthy eating plan is one of the most challenging aspects of living with diabetes. The key is to find ways to keep motivated and overcome potential hurdles:

Financial concerns. Buying lots of fresh fruits and vegetables can be expensive. But keep in mind that you're probably buying fewer less nutritious foods, such as chips and sweets. You also may be buying less meat. This saves you money.

Cultural barriers. From burritos to jambalaya to fry bread, food is an expression of culture — and no one wants to sacrifice that. But all cuisine can be prepared in healthier ways. You can find diabetic cookbooks that focus on foods from different cultures and ethnicities. These books contain plenty of ideas for making traditional foods more healthy.

Family issues. Food is often the center of social and family life. Sometimes family members aren't supportive of the changes you're trying to make. A family member may feel rejected if you say no to his or her special dish. Discuss your diabetes and treatment goals with family members and ask them for their support. Reassure family members that you're not rejecting them, just unhealthy food choices.

Social pressure. It's hard to turn down a dessert or snack when it's offered to you. If you're watching football with the guys and everyone's drinking beer and eating potato chips, it can be hard to resist. The best way to deal with potentially difficult situations is to anticipate them and plan for them. You may want to plan ahead of time how to eat a favorite dish without totally abandoning your diet plan. Another option is to bring your own healthier snacks to get-togethers, with some to share. Think through what you will eat and drink before you arrive, and stick to your plan.

Ultimately, the motivation you need to succeed will come from within. You have to believe that what you're doing matters — and you're worth it.

Rewards of staying on plan

Motivation to stick with your diet plan will improve as you begin to experience the benefits of your hard work:

You'll feel better. When you eat too much at once, or eat too many carbohydrates, your blood sugar can rise quite high. This may cause you to feel tired and fatigued. When you eat in a healthy manner, you feel better.

You'll experience fewer episodes of low blood sugar. When you skip meals or don't eat the right foods, you may experience low blood sugar (hypoglycemia). Symptoms of low blood sugar include sweating, shakiness, weakness, dizziness and irritability. Severe low blood sugar can lead to diabetic coma. Following a regular eating schedule and meal plan reduces this risk.

You'll be better able to control your weight. With an eating plan, you're less likely to overeat or eat too much of the wrong foods. Being overweight makes it more difficult to control your blood sugar. It also increases your risk of heart disease or stroke.

You'll feel in greater control. Knowing how various foods and eating patterns affect your blood sugar will help you feel as if you're controlling your diabetes — not it controlling you.

Questions and answers

Can I drink alcohol?
If your diabetes is well controlled, you may be able to drink a small amount of alcohol. But don't drink alcohol on an empty stomach. Have it with a meal and sip it slowly.

Research shows that among people in good control of their diabetes, a light to moderate amount of alcohol has only a minimal effect on blood sugar. According to some studies, moderate amounts of alcohol also may reduce your risk of heart disease and stroke. A moderate amount is defined as no more than two alcoholic drinks daily for men and one alcoholic drink daily for women. One drink equals one 12-ounce can of beer, one 5-ounce glass of wine or one 1-ounce shot glass of whiskey. Ask your doctor if it's OK for you to drink alcohol and how much.

If you're having trouble controlling your blood sugar or you have complications of diabetes, you should avoid alcohol. It can worsen some complications, including nerve damage, coronary artery disease and high blood pressure. Also, keep in mind that 1 ounce of alcohol counts as two fat servings, and that alcohol contains considerable calories. If you're trying to lose weight, alcohol may not be a good choice.

What if I don't always follow my diet?
First of all, realize that you're not always going to follow your eating plan exactly. No one is perfect. Some situations are especially challenging, such as holidays, special celebrations and eating at a restaurant or someone's home.

When you do eat more food than you should or make less healthy food choices, acknowledge that it happened and move forward. Don't beat yourself up over it, and don't try to skip a meal or eat less to make up for it. Just continue on with your regular meal plan.

It's when you regularly don't follow your eating plan that problems can develop. You may experience poor blood sugar control and develop complications. Your unhealthy habits will eventually catch up with you.

What should I eat if I'm sick?

If you can eat regular meals, stay with your usual meal plan. If you have a poor appetite but can handle some foods, eat toast, cereal, soup, fruit juice or milk. If you can't eat any solid foods and are taking insulin or oral medications, sip on fruit juice or sweetened beverages to replace carbohydrates missed in your meals.

Will vitamins or herbal supplements help me control my diabetes?

If you're eating a nutritious diet with a variety of fruits, vegetables and grains every day, you're probably getting the vitamins you need.

There's some evidence that antioxidant supplements, such as vitamins E and C, may benefit people with diabetes. The herb ginseng also may hold promise in helping some people lower their blood sugar. But not enough scientific data is available to recommend the use of vitamins and supplements for help in controlling diabetes.

Check with your doctor before taking a vitamin or herbal supplement. Some herbs may interact poorly with diabetes medications.

What about beverages or candies made from artificial sweeteners? Can I drink or eat them in unlimited amounts?

Most beverages and some hard candies that contain artificial sweeteners have almost no calories, and you can drink or eat them as often as you like. They don't count as a carbohydrate, a fat or any other exchange. Artificial sweeteners include:

- Saccharin (Sprinkle Sweet, Sweet-10, Sugar Twin, Sweet'n Low)
- Aspartame (NutraSweet, Equal)
- Acesulfame potassium (Sweet One)

Keep in mind, though, that some foods containing artificial sweeteners, such as sugar-free yogurt, may still contain calories and carbohydrates that may affect your blood sugar level.

Chapter 5

Getting more active

Our bodies are designed to move, even if modern society has made it easy to do anything but that. You may sit at a desk or in front of a computer all day and then come home and watch TV or put your feet up and read. It takes a special effort to incorporate exercise and physical activity into your day. But that effort is worth it. Exercise and increased activity bring a bounty of health benefits — especially if you have diabetes.

The information in this chapter can help you get started on the road to a more active life. You don't have to knock yourself out to reap the benefits of activity. For most people with diabetes, a moderate amount of exercise can improve their fitness and help control their disease. Even if you've never exercised before, you'll benefit from being more active.

First, a word about definitions. Physical activity is any body movement that burns calories, such as mowing the lawn, making the bed or walking up stairs. Exercise also burns calories, but it follows a planned series of repetitive movements designed to strengthen or develop all or part of your body. Exercise includes walking, swimming, bicycling and many other activities. Both physical activity and exercise are valuable to your health.

Benefits of exercise

When you exercise regularly, you:

- Improve your overall fitness, which makes it easier to do everyday activities
- Are less tired
- Improve flexibility in your muscles and joints
- Improve your muscle tone
- Improve your appearance and sense of well-being
- Reduce stress and tension
- Improve your concentration
- Increase your self-esteem
- Decrease your appetite
- Prevent bone loss and osteoporosis

These factors alone are reason enough to become more active. But for people with diabetes, the benefits of regular exercise are even greater.

Improves blood sugar control

As your muscles contract and relax during exercise, they use sugar (glucose) for energy. To meet this energy need, sugar is removed from your blood during and after exercise. This lowers your blood sugar level. Exercise also reduces blood sugar by increasing your sensitivity to insulin: Your body requires less insulin to escort sugar into your cells.

Along with a healthy eating plan, regular exercise can reduce your need for glucose-lowering medication. Some people manage their diabetes through diet and exercise alone.

In certain circumstances, exercise has the opposite effect: It can raise your blood sugar level. This usually happens if your blood sugar is greater than 300 milligrams of glucose per deciliter of blood (mg/dL) when you begin to exercise. When blood sugar is very high, exercise causes your body to release or produce extra

Are you fit?

If you sit most of the day and get little physical activity, chances are you're not fit. Other signs that you could benefit from increased physical activity and exercise include:

- Feeling tired most of the time
- Being unable to keep up with others your age
- Avoiding physical activity because you tire easily
- Becoming short of breath or fatigued when walking a short distance or up one flight of stairs

glucose. Not enough insulin is available to transport the added sugar to your cells, raising your blood sugar level.

Reduces risk of heart disease

Exercise is good for your heart and blood vessels. It improves the flow of blood through small blood vessels and increases your heart's pumping power. In combination with a healthy diet, exercise also reduces low-density lipoprotein (LDL) cholesterol, the "bad" type which causes formation of plaque in your blood vessels. In addition, exercise increases high-density lipoprotein (HDL) cholesterol — the "good" type that helps keep your arteries clean — and it helps lower blood pressure.

Controls your weight

Exercise helps you lose weight and maintain a healthy weight. Regular exercise takes off pounds by burning calories and increasing your metabolism. Exercise also helps reduce resistance to insulin that occurs from being overweight, improving your body's ability to use insulin and lowering your blood sugar level.

What type of exercise?

Aerobic exercise provides benefits for all people, including people with diabetes. Aerobic means "with oxygen." An activity is aerobic if it places added demands on your heart, lungs and muscles, increasing your breathing and heart rate and requiring increased transport of oxygen from your lungs to your circulatory system and muscles.

Aerobic activities should make up the core of your exercise program. These include activities such as:

- Walking
- Jogging
- Bicycling
- Aerobic dance
- Cross-country skiing

- Hiking
- Skating
- Golfing (walking, not riding)
- Tennis
- Swimming

Keep in mind that aerobic activities are endurance activities that don't require excessive speed. You generally benefit more from the amount of time you spend doing them than the speed at which you do them.

Take a walk

Walking is one of the easiest ways to get aerobic exercise. You don't need equipment. You don't have to learn special techniques. It's safe and inexpensive. You can walk alone or with others, indoors or outdoors.

Guidelines published by the American Association of Clinical Endocrinologists note that walking just 40 minutes four times a week is enough to lower insulin resistance, improving blood sugar control. Researchers at the Harvard School of Public Health also found that 1 hour a day of brisk walking can cut a woman's risk of developing type 2 diabetes in half.

Developing a complete fitness program

Aerobic exercise is just one component of physical fitness. Stretching and strengthening exercises also are important for good health.

Stretching exercises. Stretching before and after aerobic activity increases the range to which you can bend and stretch your joints, muscles and ligaments. Stretching exercises also help prevent joint pain and injury. The stretches should be slow and gentle. Stretch only until you feel slight tension in the muscles.

Here are four stretches you can try. Begin with 5 repetitions of each and try to build to 25 repetitions.

Calf stretch. Stand at arm's length from the wall. Lean your upper body into the wall. Place one leg forward with knee bent. Keep your other leg back with your knee straight and your heel down. Keeping your back straight, move your hips toward the wall until you feel a stretch. Hold for 30 seconds. Relax. Repeat with the other leg.

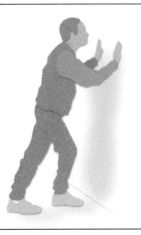

Calf stretch

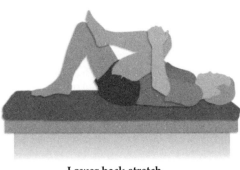

Lower back stretch

Lower back stretch. Lie on a table or bed with your hips and knees bent and your feet flat on the surface. Gently pull one knee toward your shoulder with both hands. Hold for 30 seconds. Relax. Repeat with the other leg.

Upper thigh stretch. Lie on your back on a table or a bed, with one leg and hip as near the edge as possible. Let your lower leg hang over the edge. Grasp the knee of the other leg and pull your thigh and knee firmly toward your chest until your lower back flattens against the table or

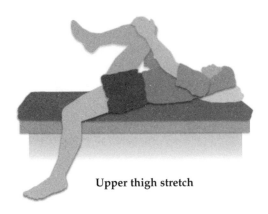

Upper thigh stretch

bed. Hold for 30 seconds. Relax. Repeat with the other leg.

Chest stretch. Clasp your hands behind your head. Pull your elbows firmly back while inhaling and exhaling deeply. Hold for 30 seconds. Relax.

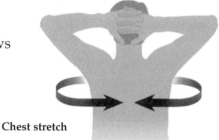

Chest stretch

Strengthening exercises. Strengthening exercises build stronger muscles to improve posture, balance and coordination. They also promote healthy bones, and they increase your rate of metabolism slightly, which can help keep your weight in check.

Here are four strengthening exercises you can try. Start with 5 repetitions of each and try to build to 25 repetitions.

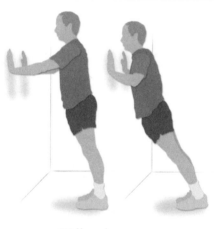

Wall push-ups

Wall push-ups. Face the wall and stand far enough away so that you can place your palms on the wall and your elbows are slightly bent. Slowly bend your elbows and lean toward the wall, supporting your weight with your arms. Straighten your arms and return to your starting position. As you build strength, try standing farther away from the wall.

Standing squats. Stand next to a table or counter with your feet slightly more than shoulder-width apart and your palms on the table or counter. Keeping your back straight, slowly bend your knees anywhere from 30 to 60 degrees. Pause and then return to your starting position.

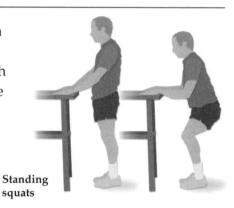

Standing squats

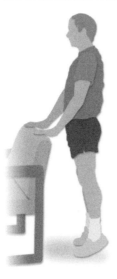

Heel raises. Stand with your feet about 12 inches apart, holding on to the back of a sturdy chair. Slowly raise your heels from the floor and stand on your tiptoes. Hold. Slowly return to the starting position.

Heel raises

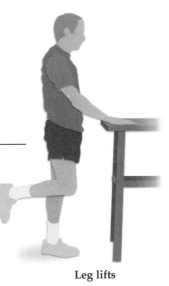

Leg lifts. Stand with your feet about 12 inches apart, holding on to a table or the back of a chair. Slowly bend one knee, lifting up your foot behind you. Hold the position, then slowly lower your leg all the way down. Repeat with the other leg.

Leg lifts

How much exercise?

You don't have to spend hours pounding the pavement or working out at a gym to benefit from exercise. Aim for at least 30 minutes of aerobic activity most days of the week.

If you haven't been active for a long time, start slowly and build up your endurance. Begin by exercising 10 minutes a day. Each week, increase the length of time you exercise by 5 minutes, and keep adding increments.

To improve your total fitness, stretch a few minutes after aerobic exercise to increase flexibility in your muscles. In addition, a couple of days a week combine your aerobic activity with some strengthening exercises. If you don't have 30 minutes or more to exercise, break your routine into shorter intervals. You might ride a stationary bicycle for 10 to 15 minutes in the morning before going to work, walk for 10 to 15 minutes during your lunch hour and do strengthening exercises for 10 to 15 minutes in the evening.

Getting started

Before you begin a fitness program, see your doctor for a thorough medical examination. Your fitness plan should be tailored to your individual physical condition and health needs. Once you have the go-ahead from your doctor and understand any limitations you may need to observe, it's time to think about what activities you want to include in your fitness program.

Select activities you enjoy

Choose a form of exercise that fits your interests. If you like the outdoors or solitude, walking or bicycling may be good choices. If you prefer being around others, you might enjoy an aerobics class or a golf group. If you prefer watching television or listening to music or books on tape while you work out, a stationary bicycle or treadmill may be options to consider.

Also keep in mind that if you have complications from your diabetes, certain types of exercise may not be good choices. For example, if you've lost feeling in your feet, swimming is better than jogging or walking. If you have trouble seeing or experience frequent episodes of low blood sugar, it may be best to exercise indoors or with a friend.

Schedule your exercise

Set aside time in your day for exercise. Write it down on your calendar or to-do list. You're more likely to make exercise a part of your daily routine if you do it at the same time each day instead of "whenever I have time." Of course, occasionally you'll need to reschedule or miss your exercise appointment, such as when you're sick or away from home. Skipping exercise to watch television, however, isn't a good excuse.

Set goals and track your progress
It's helpful to set goals because reaching a goal gives you encouragement. The key is to set goals that are specific and realistic. If you set a goal that's not attainable within a fairly short time, you'll be discouraged. Instead of starting out with a goal of jogging for 45 minutes 5 days a week, begin with a goal of walking for 20 minutes three times a week. Once you've reached that one, you can move on to a new, more challenging goal. Consider keeping a log of your progress. An exercise log helps you see what you've accomplished and determine your goals for the future.

Common excuses: Can you relate?

If you've never exercised before, or you hate to exercise, getting started on an exercise routine can be difficult. Perhaps you've used one or more of the following excuses in the past:

I'm too busy. In our increasingly hectic society, finding time to exercise can be difficult. If you can't manage 30 minutes at a time, break your exercise time into smaller parts, for example, three 10-minute intervals during the day. If you really want to improve your health, you can find the time.

I'm too old. You're never too old to exercise. Exercise provides benefits at all ages and may prevent or delay diseases as you get older. If you feel out of place at a health club, see if your local YMCA, YWCA or senior center offers exercise classes.

I'm too fat. Athletes may appear slim, trim and toned. But if you look around, you'll see that few people who exercise have a perfect physique. Walkers, bicyclers and golfers come in all shapes and sizes.

I'm too weak. You can start slowly and gradually increase your level of activity. The more you do, the stronger you'll begin to feel.

I'm too sick. You don't want to exercise if your blood sugar is out of control. But simply having diabetes isn't a reason to avoid exercise. Just the opposite, it's a reason to exercise. With time, you'll find that you'll feel less sickly.

Vary your routine

Next to lack of motivation, boredom probably kills more exercise programs than anything else does. You can keep things interesting by varying your activities. You might ride a bicycle one day, walk the next and swim another day. Choose activities that are convenient and fit with your lifestyle. Include activities for all times and seasons — when you're feeling energetic, when you're not feeling as strong, when the weather is good and when it's poor.

Finding the right intensity level

Intensity refers to how hard you work when you exercise. Exercise doesn't have to be strenuous to be of benefit. You can increase your fitness with low to moderately intense physical activities. Here are three ways to determine if you're exercising at the right intensity level. It's always a good idea to warm up before aerobic exercise and cool down afterward so that your body can gradually adjust to the changes in your activity level.

Heart rate

The harder you exercise, the higher your heart rate (pulse) climbs, until a maximum heart rate is reached. Most people should exercise at a level equivalent to 50 percent to 80 percent of their maximum heart rate. This is called your target heart rate.

In general, your target heart rate should be approxi-

Target heart rate		
Age (Years)	**Average rate (BPM)***	**Target rate (BPM)***
20	100-150	200
25	98-146	195
30	95-142	190
35	93-138	185
40	90-135	180
45	88-131	175
50	85-127	170
55	83-123	165
60	80-120	160
65	78-116	155
70	75-113	150

*BPM, beats per mintue.

mately 220 beats per minute, minus your age. To determine your heart rate, place two fingers on the side of your wrist, press gently and feel for your pulse. Count your pulse for 10 seconds and multiply the number you get by six.

Perceived exertion

Another way to gauge the intensity of your exercise routine is to use the perceived exertion scale. Perceived exertion is the total amount of physical effort you experience during a physical activity, taking into account all sensations of exertion, physical stress and fatigue.

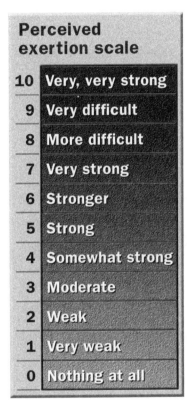

Perceived exertion scale

10	Very, very strong
9	Very difficult
8	More difficult
7	Very strong
6	Stronger
5	Strong
4	Somewhat strong
3	Moderate
2	Weak
1	Very weak
0	Nothing at all

For an activity to produce health benefits, you need to exert a moderate to somewhat strong effort. That equates to a 3 or 4 on the perceived exertion scale. A 0 rating indicates no exertion, such as when you're sitting comfortably in a chair. A 10 corresponds to maximum effort, as when jogging up a steep hill.

Talk test

While you're exercising, you should be able to carry on a short conversation without being short of breath. If you can't do this, you're probably pushing too hard and you need to slow down your pace. High-intensity exercise doesn't provide many additional fitness benefits, and it increases your risk of muscle or joint soreness and injury.

Every move counts

Regular exercise provides the greatest reward for your efforts, but you also can enjoy health benefits simply by moving around more during the day. Activities such as climbing stairs, gardening, mowing the lawn and housework help lower your blood sugar, as well as your blood cholesterol and blood pressure.

Look for ways to build more activity into your day:

- Get up to change channels on the television instead of using the remote control.
- Wash your car instead of taking it to the car wash.
- Walk or bike to the store instead of driving.
- Take the stairs instead of the elevator.
- Park farther from work and walk.
- Avoid drive-throughs. Park the car and walk.
- Weed your flower garden.
- Sweep the floors, patio and front walk.
- Prune the bushes.

Avoiding injury

As you become more active, it's important not to forget about safety.

Wear proper clothing and shoes

Select clothes that are right for the weather and your sport. Activity increases your body temperature, so it's better to underdress than to overdress. In cool weather, dress in layers so that you can remove or replace layers as you warm up or cool down. In warm weather, wear lightweight, light-colored clothes. Sweating more won't help you lose fat, just water weight, which increases your risk of overheating. Use sunscreen and wear a hat.

Make sure your shoes fit well and aren't too tight. Replace them when they begin to show signs of wear. Always put on clean, smooth-fitting socks.

Examine your feet

Check your feet before you exercise. If you see any signs of irritation, cushion the area. If you see any cuts, wash them with soap and water, treat them with an antibiotic ointment and bandage them. After you exercise, check your feet again. Look for blisters, warm areas or redness.

Drink plenty of fluids

You lose fluid when you sweat, and it's important to replace this fluid. Water is the best choice. But if you're exercising for a long period, you may want the calories and electrolytes found in sports drinks. Drink fluids before, during and after exercise. The hotter the weather, the more important it is to keep your body hydrated. Don't wait until you're thirsty to have a drink.

Pay attention to your environment

Extreme temperatures can stress your body. On hot days, exercise indoors or during the morning or evening. In general don't exercise outside if the temperature is higher than 80 F (27 C), especially if the humidity is high. Also avoid extremely cold temperatures.

Warm up and cool down

Before you begin exercising, get your body ready. Begin the exercise at a low intensity level and gradually increase the intensity level. For example, before you begin jogging or walking fast, walk for a few minutes at a slow or moderate pace to gradually increase your heart rate and oxygen flow in your lungs.

The same applies when you finish exercising, walk slowly for awhile to allow your heart rate to gradually slow down. A couple of slow stretches afterward can help keep your muscles limber and prevent them from tightening up.

Heed warning signs

No matter what your workout routine, don't ignore symptoms that may signal a problem:

- Dizziness or faintness
- Feeling sick to your stomach
- Tightness in your chest
- Severe shortness of breath
- Chest pains
- Pain in an arm or your jaw
- Heart palpitations

Exercise and blood sugar monitoring

When you first begin to exercise, it's important that you check your blood sugar often. Exercise typically reduces your blood sugar level. You want to make sure that your blood sugar isn't too low before you begin exercising and that it doesn't drop too low during and after exercise. Your blood sugar may continue to drop for a number of hours following your activity, because exercise draws on reserve sugar stored in your muscles and liver. As your body rebuilds those stores, it takes sugar from your blood, reducing your blood sugar level.

Also, remember that in some cases exercise can raise your blood sugar level. This most often occurs if your blood sugar is greater than 300 mg/dL before you begin. If your blood sugar is already high, the extra sugar can push your level into the danger zone.

To avoid low or high blood sugar levels, follow these guidelines:

Check your blood sugar twice before exercising. Test your blood sugar approximately 30 minutes before you exercise and then again right before you start. This will help you to know if your blood sugar level is stable, rising or dropping.

For most people, a safe pre-exercise blood sugar range is 100 to 250 mg/dL. If your blood sugar is under 100 mg/dL, eat a carbohydrate-containing snack to avoid having low blood sugar (hypoglycemia) while you exercise. If you have type 1 diabetes and your blood sugar level before exercising is 250 mg/dL or higher, test your urine for ketones. If the result indicates a moderate or high ketone level, don't exercise. Wait until your ketones test indicates a low level. No matter what type of diabetes you have, if your blood sugar level is more than 300 mg/dL, don't exercise. You need to bring your blood sugar down before you can safely exercise.

Check your blood sugar during exercise. This is especially important when you're trying a new activity or sport, or if you're increasing the intensity or duration of your activity. If you exercise for more than an hour, especially if you have type 1 diabetes, stop and test your blood sugar every 30 minutes. If it starts to fall, have a snack.

If you begin to experience symptoms of hypoglycemia, stop immediately and test your blood sugar. If it's low, eat something with sugar. Always carry juice, a nondiet soft drink, raisins, glucose tablets or another fast-acting source of sugar with you.

Check your blood sugar at least twice after exercise. The more strenuous your workout, the longer your blood sugar is affected following the activity. Until you have a good idea of how your body reacts to exercise, check your blood sugar frequently after your activity. Hypoglycemia also can occur hours after exercise.

Be patient

Try not to get discouraged if exercise causes significant changes in your blood sugar, interfering with your normal management routine. Continue to test your blood sugar until you begin to notice a pattern and can adjust your meals and medications accordingly. And don't be frightened off by intensive monitoring that may be required when you start exercising. As you develop a routine, you'll have a good idea of how your blood sugar will respond, and you may not need to check it as often.

Eating and exercise

The best time to exercise depends on your treatment. If you take insulin, avoid exercise 3 hours after injecting short-acting insulin due to the potential risk of low blood sugar. Both insulin and exercise lower your blood sugar. Ask your doctor what would be the best time to exercise and follow simple precautions, such as monitoring your blood sugar before you begin and carrying sugar sources with you to treat symptoms of low blood sugar. People with type 1 diabetes who exercise for more than an hour or do strenuous activities also may benefit from a snack before they begin or while exercising.

For most people with type 2 diabetes, a snack before exercise generally isn't necessary. If you don't take medications to control your diabetes, it also may be OK to exercise after you eat, when your blood sugar level is generally highest.

Questions and answers

What if I have a lapse in my routine?

It happens to everyone. You're swamped with work, on vacation or sick, and your exercise plan flies out the window. Everyone who follows a long-term exercise program has off days. Don't be too critical — remind yourself it's only a temporary setback. As soon as possible, try to resume your regular exercise schedule.

What if I don't feel like exercising?

There will be days when that will happen. Maybe you had a hard day at work, or you're dead tired or just not in the mood. On these days, try the 5-minute compromise. Tell yourself that you'll exercise for just 5 minutes. If you don't feel like continuing after 5 minutes, you can stop and not feel guilty about it. Nine times out of 10, once you've started, you'll want to continue.

Can I drink alcohol and exercise?

When you mix alcohol and exercise, you increase your risk of low blood sugar. Exercise and alcohol both tend to lower blood sugar. It's best not to drink alcohol during or after exercise. If you do, have some food with your drink.

If I'm active on my job, do I need an exercise program?

If your job is truly active — you're constantly moving 8 to 10 hours a day — it certainly counts as exercise. However, work-related activity generally doesn't offer the same intensity, relaxation level and stress-reducing benefits of exercise.

Chapter 6

Achieving a healthy weight

Being overweight is by far the greatest risk factor for type 2 diabetes. Between 80 percent and 90 percent of people who develop this type of diabetes are overweight. By contrast, most people with type 1 diabetes are at or below their ideal weight.

Why is weight such an important factor? Fat alters how your body cells respond to the hormone insulin. It causes them to become more resistant to insulin's effects, reducing the amount of sugar (glucose) the hormone is able to transport from your blood to your cells. More sugar remains in your bloodstream, increasing your blood sugar level.

The good news is that you can reverse this process. As you lose weight, your cells become more responsive to insulin, allowing it to do its job. For some people with type 2 diabetes, losing weight is all that's necessary to control their diabetes and return their blood sugar to normal. And the amount of weight loss doesn't have to be extreme. A modest weight loss of 10 to 20 pounds, or 5 percent to 10 percent of your weight, can lower your blood sugar level, as well as reduce your blood pressure and blood cholesterol levels.

Losing weight, as you well may know, can be a challenge. We believe, however, that with a positive attitude and the right advice, it's a challenge you can meet. As you develop more healthy habits, the pounds will gradually come off.

Do you need to lose weight?

Before figuring out if you're overweight by medical standards, keep in mind that what you see in the media isn't representative of typical body shapes. Many fashion models and celebrities are unrealistically thin, and you shouldn't expect to look like them. Your goal is to achieve a healthy weight — one that improves your blood sugar control and reduces your risk of other medical problems.

The three do-it-yourself evaluations that follow can tell you if your weight is healthy or whether you could benefit from weight loss.

Body mass index

Body mass index (BMI) is a measurement based on a formula that takes into account your weight and your height in determining whether you have a healthy or unhealthy percentage of body fat.

To determine your BMI, locate your height on the chart on the next page and follow that row across until you reach the column with the weight nearest yours. Look at the top of that column for the corresponding BMI rating. If your weight is less than the weight nearest yours, your BMI may be slightly less. If your weight is greater than the weight nearest yours, your BMI may be slightly greater. A BMI of 19 to 24 is considered healthy. A BMI of 25 to 29 signifies being overweight, and a BMI of 30 or more indicates obesity.

Waist circumference

Another way of determining if you're at a healthy weight is to measure your waist circumference. People who carry most of their weight around their waist often are referred to as apples. Those who carry most of their weight below the waist, around their hips and thighs, are called pears, because of their overall body shape. Generally, it's better to have a pear shape than an apple shape. That's because excess fat around your abdomen is often associated with greater risk of a heart attack and other weight-related diseases.

To determine whether you're carrying too much weight around your abdomen, measure your waist circumference at its smallest point, usually at the level of your navel. A measurement of more than 40 inches (102 centimeters) in men and 35 inches (88 centimeters) in women signifies increased health risks, especially if you have a BMI of 25 to 35.

BMI	HEALTHY		OVERWEIGHT		OBESE			
	19	24	25	29	30	35	40	45
HEIGHT	WEIGHT IN POUNDS							
4'10"	91	115	119	138	143	167	191	215
4'11"	94	119	124	143	148	173	198	222
5'0"	97	123	128	148	153	179	204	230
5'1"	100	127	132	153	158	185	211	238
5'2"	104	131	136	158	164	191	218	246
5'3"	107	135	141	163	169	197	225	254
5'4"	110	140	145	169	174	204	232	262
5'5"	114	144	150	174	180	210	240	270
5'6"	118	148	155	179	186	216	247	278
5'7"	121	153	159	185	191	223	255	287
5'8"	125	158	164	190	197	230	262	295
5'9"	128	162	169	196	203	236	270	304
5'10"	132	167	174	202	209	243	278	313
5'11"	136	172	179	208	215	250	286	322
6'0"	140	177	184	213	221	258	294	331
6'1"	144	182	189	219	227	265	302	340
6'2"	148	186	194	225	233	272	311	350
6'3"	152	192	200	232	240	279	319	359
6'4"	156	197	205	238	246	287	328	369

Personal and family history

An evaluation of your medical history, along with that of your family, is equally important in determining if your weight is healthy.

- Do you have a health condition that would benefit from weight loss? For most people with type 2 diabetes, the answer to this question is yes.

- Do you have a family history of a weight-related illness, such as diabetes or high blood pressure?

- Have you gained considerable weight since high school? Weight gain in adulthood is associated with increased health risks.

- Do you smoke cigarettes, have more than two alcoholic drinks a day or live with considerable stress? In combination with these behaviors, excess weight can have greater health implications.

Your results

If your BMI shows that you aren't overweight and you're not carrying too much weight around your abdomen, there's probably no health advantage to changing your weight. Your weight is healthy.

If your BMI is between 25 and 29 or your waist circumference exceeds healthy guidelines, you could probably benefit from losing a few pounds, especially if you answered yes to at least one personal and family health question. Discuss your weight with your doctor during your next checkup.

If your BMI is 30 or more, losing weight will improve your overall health and reduce your risk of future illness, including complications of diabetes.

Healthy weight loss

Eating sensibly and keeping active are the keys to successful weight loss. But putting these practices to work can be more difficult than it seems. Our society is set up in a way that makes it easy to gain weight, not lose it. We ride in cars, take elevators, use an array of labor-saving devices and spend hours in front of the computer and the television. High-calorie foods are widely available, and fatty foods taste good. We're bombarded with commercial messages urging us to eat, and large portions are the norm.

To lose weight you have to go against the grain. You have to be willing to change your habits. And there's no magic bullet or quick fix to help you out. No matter how much you hear about diet supplements or trendy diet plans, the human body can't defy the laws of nature. To lose weight you have to expend more energy than you take in, which means eating fewer calories and moving more.

Sound boring? Not if you have the right attitude. Rather than saying you're dieting, view your efforts as a lifestyle improvement. And don't focus only on the end result — enjoy the process of getting there.

All those fad diets

Fad diets have been around for decades and new ones emerge every year. Some of the most popular diets, such as the Atkins diet and the Zone diet, limit consumption of carbohydrates on the theory that carbohydrates promote insulin production, which leads to weight gain.

Carbohydrates eaten in reasonable quantities don't cause increased insulin levels, as many of these diets claim. The reason these diets work for some people is simply because the diets limit the total number of calories, sometimes excessively. The trouble is, most people can only stick with fad diets for a short while before they go off them and eventually gain their weight back. In addition, very low-calorie diets are unhealthy. They generally include few grains, fruits and vegetables, which provide numerous vitamins and minerals and help prevent disease. Without these essential carbohydrates, your body begins to burn glycogen and fat for energy, producing ketones. This can be dangerous for people with diabetes.

In general, the negatives of fad diets outweigh the positives.

Are you ready?

No one can make you lose weight. In fact, pressure from others only makes matters worse. You must be internally motivated to lose weight because it's what you want.

But that doesn't mean that you have to do it all alone. Your doctor or a registered dietitian can help you develop a plan to lose weight. You can ask for support from your spouse, family and friends. You may even want to join a support group, such as Weight Watchers or Take Off Pounds Sensibly (TOPS).

To help determine if you're ready to change your eating and exercise habits, ask yourself the following questions:

- *How motivated do I feel to make lifestyle changes now?* Be honest. Knowing that you need to make changes and feeling up to the challenge are two different things.

- *What's going on in my life right now?* If you've just been diagnosed with a health condition, such as diabetes, now may be the right time to lose weight. Your thoughts and energies are focused on improving your health.

- *Do I have time to keep track of what I eat and how much I exercise?* Studies show that keeping food and exercise records increases your chance of success.

- *Do I truly believe that I can change my eating behavior?* To be successful, you have to believe that you can change.

- *Am I willing to find ways to be more physically active?* Weight loss isn't just about what you eat. Exercise is an important part of the process.

- *Can I view this as a positive, even pleasurable, experience?* If you can take pleasure in what you're doing, your chances of being successful are greatly improved.

Do you have a 'dieter's mentality'?

A "dieter's mentality" sets you up to fail. Instead of making permanent changes in your eating habits, you're always waiting until you can go off your diet and eat the way you'd like. Do any of these attitudes sound familiar?

- There are good foods and bad foods.
- I'm either on a diet or off.
- If I eat something I like, then I'm cheating.
- Staying on my diet takes a lot of willpower.
- Being on a diet means always being hungry.
- If I have a setback, I'm a failure.

Achieving and maintaining a healthy weight requires a permanent change in your lifestyle. Instead of using the "D" word, find a positive phrase that reflects the changes you're making, such as "I'm improving my eating and exercise habits," or "I'm paying more attention to my health."

Set realistic goals

Losing weight is often easier when you have a goal to strive for. But it's important that you start small. If your goal is to lose 50 pounds within a year, break it down into smaller goals. Your first goal might be to lose 3 to 4 pounds within a month. Once you achieve that goal, set a new one. Another goal might be to increase your daily servings of fruits and vegetables.

Plan also for how you're going to achieve your goals — losing those 3 to 4 pounds or eating more fruits and vegetables. You might make it a goal to walk for 30 minutes 5 days a week or to try a new recipe each week that contains fruit or vegetables.

Follow your healthy eating plan

If you've developed an eating plan to manage your diabetes, you're one step ahead of many people who are trying to lose weight. The same eating plan for controlling your blood sugar discussed in Chapter 4 also can help you lose weight, as long as you pay attention to the total amount of calories you consume each day.

A dietitian can help you determine a daily calorie goal to help you lose weight. He or she takes into account a variety of factors, including your weight, sex, activity level, age, height and overall health. If you're a woman and weigh less than 250 pounds, your calorie goal may fall between 1,200 and 1,400 calories each day. If you're a man and weigh less than 250 pounds, your daily goal may be between 1,400 and 1,600 calories. These calorie amounts may seem restrictive, but they take into account that most people consume more calories each day than they think they do. If you weigh more than 250 pounds, your calorie goal will be higher.

For many people, simply replacing a few servings of fats, dairy products or meat with lower-calorie fruits, vegetables and grains is enough to reach their calorie goal. Small changes also add up. For example, by switching from whole milk to skim milk, you save 60 calories a cup. If you drink a cup of milk each day, that's 420 calories a week.

Eating less than your calorie goal generally isn't recommended because you aren't able to eat enough food to keep you satisfied, and you're soon hungry again. Eating fewer than 1,200 to 1,400 calories also can make it difficult to get enough of certain nutrients you need for good health.

Keep a food record

Research shows that people who record the foods they eat each day often are more successful at weight loss than those who don't keep track. For one thing, most people underestimate the number of calories they eat by at least 20 percent. Each day, write down everything you eat.

You might also start a food journal. A food journal simply is an expansion of a food record. In addition to recording what you eat, you include information on when and where you eat, whether you're hungry, and your mood or feelings when you eat. You may find that certain feelings trigger particular eating behaviors. Maybe you overeat when you're depressed, angry or sad. Or maybe you eat when you're bored, even if you're not hungry.

Review your food record or food journal weekly to identify potential problems or barriers to success.

Identify your unique challenges

Knowing your food triggers can help you improve your eating habits. Maybe your problem isn't using food to relieve your feelings, but your simple love of particular foods, such as ice cream or salty snacks. Or perhaps you have a compulsive need to clean your plate.

The first step in changing any habit is to become aware of it. Just admitting your bad habits won't get you past them, but it will help you plan how to deal with them. If you want to beat the odds, you need to identify the factors that lead to your being overweight, and then think about how you're going to respond differently in the future.

Here are some strategies that may work for you:

- Before eating anything, ask yourself if you're really hungry.

- When you have a craving for an unhealthy snack, distract yourself. Call a friend, take a walk or run an errand.

- Limit eating to the kitchen or dining room table. Don't allow yourself to eat in the living room or your bedroom, or while walking or standing around.

- When you eat, focus on eating. Don't watch television, read or talk on the phone.

- Store food out of sight in your cupboards or refrigerator.

- Don't keep high-calorie foods around. If it's out of the house, it's out of your mouth.

Plan for difficult situations

If you're going to be in a situation that you know will be difficult for you, such as a neighborhood or social gathering with lots of hors d'oeuvres, develop a plan of action before you go. Eat something healthy just before you leave so that so you won't be so hungry once you arrive. Decide in advance how many hors d'oeuvres you can eat. Then eat them slowly, truly savoring the flavors. If you're still hungry, head for the vegetable tray.

Get and stay active

What and how much you eat are crucial to achieving a healthy weight and good diabetes control, but food isn't the only factor. Activity is equally important. Daily exercise and increased physical activity can double your weight loss. Exercise and physical activity also are the most important factors in long-term weight loss — they'll help you keep the pounds off! For information on how to add more activity to your day, see Chapter 5.

Accept and deal with setbacks

It's inevitable that you'll have setbacks, and that's OK. But don't use your setbacks as an excuse to dump your eating and activity goals. Instead, simply continue on with your plan. If you couldn't walk today because you ran out of time, walk an extra 5 minutes the next few days. If you ate a slice of pizza that you hadn't planned on, think about what triggered you to do so and try to learn from it.

You're not going to be perfect. Reflect on your successes, and remind yourself of the reasons you want to lose weight.

Modifying recipes

Many recipes contain unnecessary amounts of fat, calories or sugar and can be modified so they're more healthy. It's more important to modify the recipes you use frequently than something you make only once a year for a special occasion.

Experiment with some of your favorite recipes to see if you can make them healthier without sabotaging their taste:

Reduce the amount of sugar or fat. The amount of sugar in most recipes can be reduced by one-third to one-half the original amount. Follow the general guideline of a quarter cup of sweetener (sugar, honey or molasses) for every cup of flour.

Fat in many baked products and casseroles also can be reduced by one-third to one-half. In baked goods substitute half the shortening with applesauce or puréed fruit. In casseroles cut the amount of meat in half or replace the meat with lentils or beans. The amount of cheese in most recipes also can be reduced by half.

Delete an ingredient. Ingredients used primarily for appearance or by habit can be eliminated. Examples include toppings such as nuts, coconut, frosting and cheese, and condiments such as ketchup, mayonnaise and jam.

Change the method of preparation. Instead of frying, use low-fat cooking methods, such as baking, broiling, grilling, poaching or steaming.

Reduce your serving size. By eating half a serving, you consume only half the calories, sugar and fat.

Questions and answers

I have a weakness for sweets. Can I still eat some and lose weight?
You can eat sweets once in a while without destroying your overall
eating plan or interfering with your blood sugar control. It's generally best to eat them with a meal, and you need to include them in
your meal plan. A dietitian can help you incorporate your favorite
treats into your meal plan. Also, many diabetic cookbooks include
tasty dessert recipes.

As you acquire new eating habits, you may find that your tastes
will change. Foods that you once loved may seem too sweet. You
may discover that a bowl of berries topped with a spoonful of fat-
free sour cream or fat-free whipping cream and a sprinkle of cinna-
mon is your new idea of delicious.

Why can't I just diet without exercising?
Most eating plans that focus solely on food aren't as successful in
the long term as those that combine a healthy diet and exercise.
Exercise helps your body burn calories more efficiently, even at rest,
helping you maintain weight loss. It also strengthens your body
and gives you energy. A downfall of some fad diets, especially
those low in carbohydrates, is fatigue.

**Aren't some fruits and vegetables high in fat and calories, such
as avocados?**
You needn't avoid any fruits and vegetables. But certain vegetables, such as corn, potatoes and peas, contain more calories and
carbohydrates than others. Many fruits also are high in calories.
Avocados are high in calories and fat.

Refer to your diabetes exchange lists or ask your dietitian about
vegetables and fruits that can be eaten in unlimited quantities and
those that you need to include in your daily meal plan.

**What about liquid diet products? Is it OK to drink them in place
of a meal if I don't have time to eat?**
Studies involving the diet product Slim Fast show that Slim Fast
doesn't negatively influence blood sugar, and when combined with

a healthy diet and regular exercise, it can lead to weight loss. Slim Fast contains all of the required daily vitamins and minerals, and it also has some fiber. A healthy diet that includes whole grains, fruits and vegetables is best, but Slim Fast is a convenient alternative when eating a healthy meal isn't possible.

Products similar to Slim Fast may provide similar benefits, but they haven't been studied.

What about prescription medications for weight loss? Can I take them if I have diabetes?

Weight loss medications available by prescription include the drugs sibutramine (Meridia) and orlistat (Xenical). Having diabetes doesn't prevent you from taking these medications. However, the drugs aren't recommended if you have certain health conditions.

Sibutramine inhibits the breakdown of serotonin and adrenaline, two substances implicated in appetite control. The drug can increase your blood pressure and shouldn't be taken if you have heart disease or uncontrolled high blood pressure, you've had a stroke, or you're taking an antidepressant. Common side effects of sibutramine include a dry mouth, headaches and insomnia.

Orlistat interferes with your body's absorption of dietary fat. It isn't recommended for people with digestive problems, including chronic malabsorption syndrome and cholestasis. Common side effects include more frequent bowel movements, passage of gas (flatulence) and diarrhea.

These medications should be used with caution and in conjunction with regular exercise and dietary changes. It's important that you discuss the potential benefits and risks of these drugs with your doctor in determining if the medications are right for you.

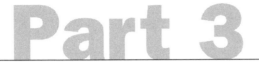

Part 3

Medical Therapies

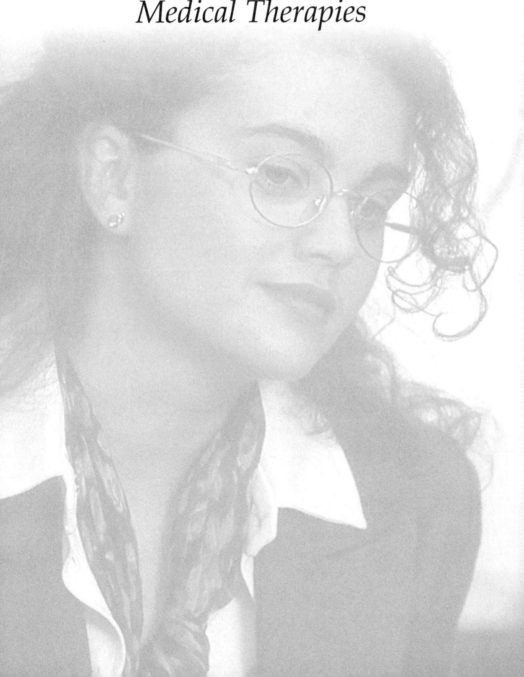

Chapter 7

Medications
for type 1 diabetes

A healthy diet and regular exercise are crucial to any diabetes treatment plan. But sometimes diet and exercise aren't enough. You need the help of medication. For people with type 1 diabetes, daily administration of the hormone insulin is essential. To live, you must supply your body with insulin medication to replace the insulin your pancreas is no longer able to produce. If you have type 2 diabetes and don't benefit from other medications, you also may need to take insulin.

Use of insulin to treat diabetes, called insulin therapy, has two main goals:

- To maintain blood sugar (glucose) at near-normal levels
- To prevent long-term complications of diabetes

A successful treatment plan takes into consideration what you eat and how much you exercise in determining the amount of insulin you need each day.

A brief history

People diagnosed with diabetes faced a bleak future well into the 20th century. Treatments were severe — some people were purposely starved to get a handle on their blood sugar levels, and others were given enormous amounts of fluid, even alcohol, to flush their system of impurities. Regardless of the treatment, most people didn't live longer than a year after their diagnosis.

Since the landmark discovery of insulin by Canadian surgeon Frederick Banting and medical student Charles Best in 1921, the outlook for people with diabetes has been remarkably brighter. Banting and Best injected the hormone into people with diabetes, causing the patients' blood sugar levels to drop and their symptoms to improve. A year later, in 1922, insulin became commercially available to the public.

But several years later, new problems emerged. People with diabetes began to develop chronic medical problems associated with damaged blood vessels and nerves, long-term effects of the disease. Instead of dying from acute complications of too little insulin, they were going blind and dying from heart and kidney disease.

For decades researchers worked to improve the purity of insulin and to develop insulin preparations with longer-lasting action in the body. Initially, the insulin used to treat diabetes came from the pancreases of cattle (bovine insulin), pigs (porcine insulin) or a combination of the two. But animal insulin has some limitations. Most forms have impurities (protein substances) that can cause allergic reactions in people who receive the insulin. The speed at which animal insulin is absorbed into your bloodstream and its effect on your cells also is different than human insulin. In addition, some people experience skin irritation at the site of the injection. For these reasons, animal insulin is less commonly used today. The most widely used form of insulin is synthetic human insulin. It's called human insulin because its chemical makeup is identical to that of insulin produced by the human pancreas, but this insulin is made in a laboratory.

Another hurdle over the years has been finding a way to mimic normal concentrations of insulin in your blood. Your pancreas releases a low-level amount of insulin throughout the day and night. Following a meal, the amount of insulin it secretes increases to control a rise in blood sugar. In just the last 20 years, the hard work of many researchers has started paying off. A variety of new tools and insulin preparations are making it possible to more closely match insulin therapy to your body's natural insulin requirements.

How insulin works

It's easier to understand the importance of insulin therapy if you understand how insulin normally works in your body. As we discussed in previous chapters, food is made up of carbohydrates, protein and fats. All three affect your blood sugar, but carbohydrates affect it the most. Carbohydrates are broken down and absorbed into your bloodstream in the form of sugar (glucose), raising your blood sugar level.

Your pancreas releases insulin continuously, whether or not you're eating. When the amount of sugar in your blood rises, however, such as after a meal, secretion of insulin increases. The main job of insulin is to keep your blood sugar level within its normal range. It does this by "escorting" sugar — your body's main energy supply — from your bloodstream to your individual cells. As sugar enters your cells, the amount of sugar in your blood drops.

Insulin also influences your liver, which plays a key role in maintaining normal blood sugar levels. After you eat, when insulin levels are high, your liver accepts and stores extra sugar in the form of glycogen. Between meals, when insulin levels are low, your liver releases glycogen into your bloodstream in the form of sugar, keeping your blood sugar level within a narrow and normal range.

Types of insulin

All people with type 1 diabetes and some people with type 2 diabetes need insulin medication to make up for the insulin that their pancreas is unable to produce. The medication is administered by injection with a syringe or an insulin pen, or through constant infusion from an insulin pump. Insulin isn't available in pill form because its chemical structure is destroyed during digestion, making the hormone ineffective by the time it gets to your bloodstream. Many types of insulin are used, and they differ in the time it takes for them to begin working and in their duration. The diagrams below show the peak action and duration of different forms of insulin. Peak action refers to the amount of time the hormone is working the hardest. The times given are approximate.

Short-acting insulin

Short-acting insulin works quickly, but its effects last for only a limited time:

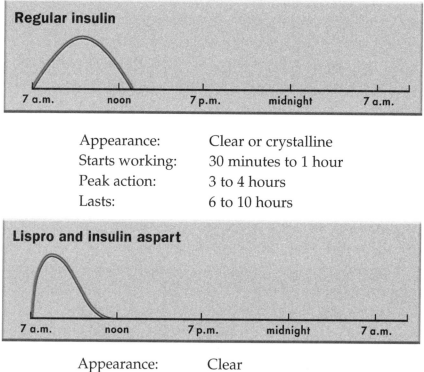

Appearance:	Clear or crystalline
Starts working:	30 minutes to 1 hour
Peak action:	3 to 4 hours
Lasts:	6 to 10 hours

Appearance:	Clear
Starts working:	Within 15 minutes
Peak action:	1 hour
Lasts:	3 to 5 hours

Intermediate-acting insulin

Intermediate-acting insulin starts working later than short-acting insulin, and its effects last longer:

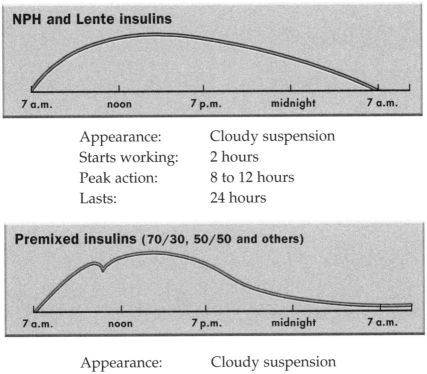

Appearance:	Cloudy suspension
Starts working:	2 hours
Peak action:	8 to 12 hours
Lasts:	24 hours

Appearance:	Cloudy suspension
Starts working:	30 minutes to 1 hour
Peak action:	3 hours and again at 8 to 12 hours
Lasts:	24 hours

Long-acting insulin

Long-acting insulin takes several hours to work, but the duration of its peak action is greater than that of other forms of insulin:

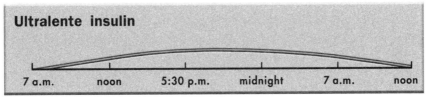

Appearance:	Cloudy suspension
Starts working:	7 hours
Peak action:	More than 22 hours
Lasts:	More than 24 hours

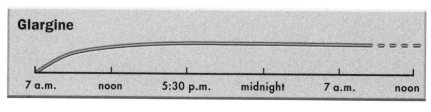

Appearance:	Clear
Starts working:	1 to 2 hours
Peak action:	Up to 24 hours
Lasts:	24 hours or longer

Insulin analogues

The goal of any insulin program is to keep blood sugar within or close to its normal range by mimicking normal pancreatic secretions of insulin. Ideally, this regimen would provide continuous (basal) secretion of insulin as well as periodic meal-related secretions. As useful as the current types of human insulin are, they're not perfect. Their action and rate of absorption vary.

Researchers have discovered that by rearranging the chemical structure of synthetic human insulin, they can create modified forms of insulin called insulin analogues. The onset and duration of these newer types of insulin more closely resemble those of natural insulin.

Lispro (Humalog) and insulin aspart (NovoLog). These forms of insulin are called rapid-acting because they're absorbed more quickly than regular insulin. They also peak faster and their effects wear off sooner. Lispro and insulin aspart work just long enough to keep your blood sugar from rising too high after meals.

One of the downfalls of rapid-acting insulins — which also can occur with other types of insulin — is that they can cause your blood sugar level to drop too low (hypoglycemia) if they're administered too early before a meal. To prevent this from occurring, these medications should be taken at the time you eat.

Glargine (Lantus). Researchers hope long-acting insulin analogues can provide more consistent blood sugar control. Development of these medications has been slow but one such insulin analogue has received Food and Drug Adminstration approval. Glargine requires only one injection a day, begins working 1 to 2 hours after injection and has no distinct peak effect.

Insulin regimens

The type and dosage of insulin you need depends on the characteristics of your disease. Your daily insulin regimen may involve one or two types of insulin. Mixing two types of insulin often can more accurately mimic normal insulin production. You might take a short-acting insulin to simulate insulin secretion at mealtime and a longer-acting insulin to mimic basal insulin secretions.

Your doctor will help you decide which insulin regimen will work best for your diabetes and your lifestyle. Several types of insulin regimens exist:

Single dose. You inject a dose of intermediate-acting insulin once each day. This regimen is the least beneficial for people with type 1 diabetes.

Mixed dose. You inject both short-acting and intermediate-acting insulins — mixed in one syringe — each morning.

Premixed single dose. You inject a dose of premixed insulin each morning.

Split dose. You give yourself two injections of intermediate-acting insulin each day. These injections are usually given before breakfast and before the evening meal, or before breakfast and at bedtime.

Split mixed dose. You give yourself two injections that contain a combination of a short-acting and an intermediate-acting insulin — mixed in one syringe — each day. These are generally given before breakfast and before the evening meal.

Split premixed dose. You give yourself two injections of premixed insulin daily. These are usually given before breakfast and before the evening meal, or before breakfast and at bedtime.

Intensive insulin therapy. This regimen involves multiple daily injections of insulin or use of a small portable pump that continuously administers insulin.

Intensive insulin therapy

One of many things researchers have learned is that people taking insulin have less risk of complications from their diabetes if they can keep their blood sugar within a normal or near-normal range — called intensive insulin therapy or tight blood sugar control. This is the preferred form of therapy for people with type 1 diabetes. It also is recommended for some people with type 2 diabetes.

Intensive insulin therapy involves monitoring your blood sugar frequently, using a combination of insulins and adjusting your insulin doses based on your blood sugar levels, your diet and changes in your routine. When practiced effectively, intensive insulin therapy can:

- Reduce your risk of eye damage
- Reduce your risk of kidney disease
- Reduce your risk of nerve damage
- Improve your cholesterol levels
- Significantly reduce your risk of heart disease

Two methods for implementing intensive insulin therapy are:

Multiple daily injections (MDIs). Multiple daily injection therapy includes three or more injections of insulin daily to achieve good blood sugar control. Both a short-acting insulin and a longer-acting insulin are used.

An insulin pump. An insulin pump most closely resembles how your body delivers insulin. The short-acting insulin used with insulin pumps offers more consistent and predictable effects than longer-acting insulin. Insulin pumps are discussed in greater detail later in this chapter.

Drawbacks of tight control

Intensive insulin therapy has two possible drawbacks: low blood sugar (hypoglycemia) and weight gain. The tighter your blood sugar levels, the greater your risk of experiencing low blood sugar when your routine changes and your blood sugar varies from its normal range. You can counter this risk by being aware of the symptoms of low blood sugar and responding quickly when you begin to experience them. For more information on low blood sugar, see Chapter 2.

Weight gain can occur because the more insulin you use to control your blood sugar, the more sugar that gets into your cells and the less sugar that's wasted in your urine. Sugar that your cells don't use accumulates as fat. Following a healthy eating plan can help limit weight gain.

Injecting insulin

When first diagnosed with diabetes, you may feel frightened or nervous about injecting yourself with insulin. That's natural. Learning about the process and doing it a few times will help you feel more comfortable. The most common way to receive insulin is by syringe. This method delivers insulin underneath the skin, where it's absorbed into the bloodstream. An alternative method for injecting insulin involves the use of an insulin pen (see "Newer injection tools" on the following page).

Selecting a site
Insulin may be injected into any area of your body where a layer of fatty tissue is present and where large blood vessels, nerves, muscles and bones aren't close to the surface. Direct injection of insulin into your bloodstream — although sometimes done in a hospital — isn't recommended for day-to-day use because it's inconvenient and would make the insulin act too fast. Insulin is absorbed most evenly from injections in the abdomen except for the 2-inch radius around the navel. Rotate the site of each injection.

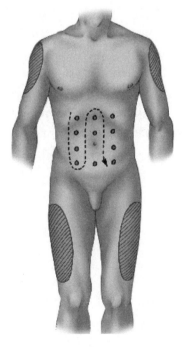

Newer injection tools

For many years a standard syringe containing a needle was the only tool used to inject insulin. Now other options are available:

Insulin pen injectors. Although a needle is still involved, insulin pens offer a convenient, more accurate and discreet means of receiving insulin. This device looks like a pen with a cartridge — but the cartridge is filled with insulin

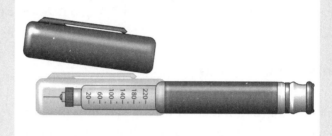

rather than ink. Some pens use disposable cartridges containing prefilled insulin. Other pens are completely disposable. You place a fine point needle, much like the one on a syringe, on the tip of the pen. You turn a dial to select the desired insulin dose, insert the needle under your skin and then click down on a button at the end of the pen to deliver the insulin.

Nondisposable pen injectors cost between $35 and $60, with additional costs for needles and insulin cartridges. Pen injectors that are completely disposable are more expensive. Although syringe needles are still the most common way to inject insulin, pens are becoming more popular.

Insulin jet injectors. These devices use high-pressure air to send a fine spray of insulin under your skin. This can be a painful way to receive insulin, and it's not as accurate as other methods because some of the medication can be lost during injection. Jet injectors may be an option if you can't use needles. However, if you use the device incorrectly, you could injure your skin. Jet injectors are more expensive than pen injectors, generally costing $250 or more.

Your doctor or diabetes educator may show you alternative areas for injection, such as your hips, buttocks, upper arms and thighs. It's generally best to administer insulin in your abdomen because insulin absorption in other areas is more variable and often dependent on your level of physical activity. After you determine the site for your insulin injection, clean it with an alcohol wipe or soap and water, and allow it to dry before giving yourself an injection.

Drawing insulin into a syringe

With time and practice the process of drawing insulin into a syringe becomes routine and is no longer so daunting. Here's how to do it:

- Collect the materials you'll need: alcohol wipes, insulin and a syringe.

- Check the label on the insulin bottle for the source, type, concentration and expiration date. You should use the same kind of insulin every time, unless your doctor tells you otherwise. Changing insulin types may affect blood sugar control.

- Check the insulin bottle for any changes in the insulin. Make sure no clumping, frosting, precipitation or change in clarity or color has occurred. Any changes in appearance may mean that the insulin has lost potency.

- Wash your hands with soap and water.

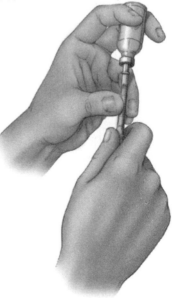

- Gently roll the bottle of insulin between your hands to mix the insulin. Shaking it may decrease its potency. Check to make sure that no particles remain on the bottom of the bottle.

- Wipe off the top of the insulin bottle with an alcohol wipe.

- Remove the needle cap from the sterile syringe.

- Pull the plunger to draw into the syringe an amount of air equal to the amount of insulin you need.

- Insert the needle through the rubber stopper of the insulin bottle and push the air in the syringe into the bottle.

- While keeping the needle in the bottle, turn the bottle completely upside down.

- Pull the plunger on the syringe slightly past the number of units of insulin you are to inject. Be sure that you're withdrawing insulin, not air. Air isn't dangerous but it can decrease the amount of insulin in the syringe.

- Remove air bubbles either by pushing the insulin back into the bottle and withdrawing it again or snapping the syringe sharply with your finger and then pushing the plunger to expel the air into the bottle.

- Recheck the syringe for air. If air is present, repeat the previous step.

- Double-check the amount of insulin in the syringe.

- Pull the needle out of the bottle.

If you need to inject two types of insulin at the same time, write on a piece of paper the amount of each type of insulin to be injected and add the two to determine the total number of units. Follow the preceding steps for drawing up insulin until you reach the point that you remove the sterile cap from the syringe. From then on, do as follows:

- Pull the plunger to draw into the syringe an amount of air equal to the amount of intermediate- or long-acting insulin you need.

- Insert the needle through the rubber stopper of the intermediate- or long-acting insulin bottle and push the air in the syringe into the bottle. This will equalize air pressure in the vial. Without it, it'll be hard to withdraw the insulin.

- Pull the needle out of the bottle *without withdrawing any insulin*.

- Pull the plunger to draw into the syringe an amount of air equal to the amount of short-acting insulin you need.

- Insert the needle through the rubber stopper on the short-acting insulin bottle and push the air in the syringe into the bottle.

- While keeping the needle in the bottle, turn the bottle completely upside down.

- Pull the plunger on the syringe slightly past the number of units of short-acting insulin you are to inject. Be sure that you're withdrawing insulin, not air.

- Remove air bubbles either by pushing the insulin back into the bottle and withdrawing it again or by snapping the syringe sharply with your finger and then pushing the plunger to expel the air into the bottle.

- Recheck the syringe for air. If air is present, repeat the previous step.

- Double-check the amount of insulin in the syringe.

- Pull the needle out of the bottle.

- Insert the needle through the rubber stopper of the intermediate- or long-acting insulin bottle.

- While keeping the needle in the bottle, turn the bottle completely upside down.

- Carefully withdraw the required number of insulin units. If you draw past the correct amount, don't push the insulin back into the bottle. Throw away the syringe and begin again.

- Double-check the amount of insulin in the syringe. It should equal the sum on your piece of paper.

- Pull the needle out of the bottle.

Injecting insulin

Once you have the right amount of insulin in the syringe and you've removed the needle from the bottle, it's time to inject the medication:

- Hold the syringe like a pencil. Quickly insert the entire length of the needle into a fold of your skin at a 90-degree angle (see illustration on the following page). If you're thin, you may need to use a short needle or inject at a 45-degree angle to avoid injecting into your muscle, especially in the thigh area.

- Release the
  pinched skin and
  inject the insulin
  by gently pushing
  the plunger all the
  way down at a
  steady, moderate
  rate. If the plunger
  jams as you're
  injecting the
  insulin, remove
  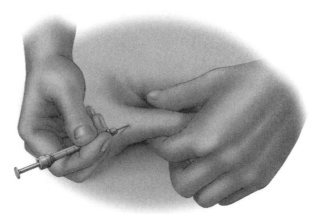
  the needle and note the number of units remaining in the
  syringe. Contact your doctor, nurse or diabetes educator for
  more instructions.

- Place the alcohol wipe on your skin next to
  the needle and withdraw the needle.

- Apply gentle pressure with the alcohol wipe at the injection
  site for 3 to 5 seconds. Don't rub.

- Discard the needle in a covered, puncture resistant container.

Preventing skin reactions

Occasionally, especially when you first start using insulin, you may
notice redness and slight swelling at the injection site. This irritation usually disappears in 2 to 3 weeks. It could be the result of
impurities in the insulin, or it could stem from a small amount of
alcohol getting into fat tissues. To avoid this, let the injection site
dry after cleaning it with alcohol. If the skin irritation lasts more
than 2 to 3 weeks or causes you discomfort, talk to your doctor.

You can minimize painful injections by doing the following:

- Make sure the insulin is at room temperature.

- Be sure no air bubbles are in the syringe.

- Relax your muscles in the area of the injection.

- Penetrate your skin quickly with the needle.

- Don't change the direction of the needle during the injection.

Avoiding potential problems

The following steps can reduce your risk of problems from insulin use:

Purchase all of your insulin from the same pharmacist. This will help ensure that you receive insulin from the same source and of the same type and concentration, unless your doctor advises a change. Check the expiration date on the package and always keep a spare bottle on hand.

Store your insulin in the refrigerator until it's opened. After a bottle has been opened, it may be kept at room temperature for 1 month. Insulin at room temperature causes less discomfort when injected. Throw away your insulin after the expiration date or after being kept at room temperature for a month.

Avoid temperature extremes. Never freeze insulin or expose it to extremely hot temperatures or direct sunlight.

Look for changes in appearance. Throw away insulin that is discolored or contains solid particles.

Wear diabetes identification. Wear an identification necklace or bracelet that identifies you as an insulin user. In addition, carry an identification card that includes the name and phone number of your doctor and all the medications you're taking, including the kind of insulin. In case your blood sugar drops too low, this will help people know how to respond.

Speak up. To avoid possible drug interactions or drug side effects, inform your dentist, pharmacist and those doctors that may not be familiar with your medical history that you take insulin.

Check all medications. Before taking any medication other than your insulin, including over-the-counter products, read the warning label. If the label says you shouldn't take the drug if you have diabetes, consult your doctor before taking it.

Some people develop indentations, hard lumps or thickened skin in areas where they inject insulin. Ask your doctor or diabetes educator what you can do to avoid this. Often, rotating the site of your injections will prevent or reduce this problem. Avoid injecting in areas of indentations, hard lumps or thickened skin because insulin isn't absorbed as well there.

In rare instances, insulin injections can cause a severe allergic reaction, including breathing and swallowing difficulties. This is a medical emergency, and you should see a doctor immediately.

Insulin pumps

In the early 1960s the notion of providing ongoing delivery of insulin first emerged. This idea led to a device called an insulin pump, which could provide a continuous supply of insulin, eliminating the need for daily shots. The first insulin pump was too cumbersome to be practical, but by the late 1970s, a portable pump evolved that offered promise. The first reported experience of using portable pumps was in London in 1978. This was followed by several studies confirming the effectiveness of pump therapy, known as continuous subcutaneous insulin infusion (CSII).

As insulin pumps have become smaller and more advanced, their use has become more widespread. Today's pumps are smaller than a deck of cards and can be hooked to a belt. Unlike earlier models, their batteries last longer and require changing only every month or two.

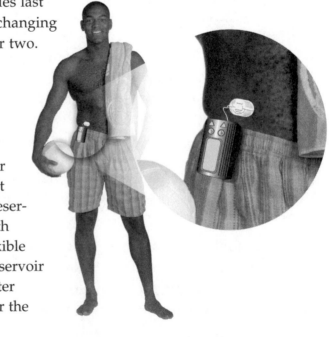

How insulin pumps work
An insulin pump is a small pumping device that you wear outside your body. It contains a syringe reservoir that you fill with insulin. A small, flexible tube connects the reservoir of insulin to a catheter that's inserted under the

skin of your abdomen. You use a needle to insert the catheter and then withdraw the needle.

The pump disperses the desired amount of insulin through the catheter into your body, based on the information you've programmed into the microprocessor. Insulin is administered continuously by slow infusion at a rate determined by your doctor. You also can program the pump to deliver larger amounts of insulin during meals, based on the amount of food you eat. This increased dose is called a bolus of insulin.

Every second or third day you need to change the infusion site. To do this, you pull out the catheter and insert a new one at a different site. Your doctor or diabetes educator will likely recommend that you rotate the injection site among the four quadrants of your abdomen. The reservoir that holds the insulin also needs to be refilled every few days.

If you decide to use an insulin pump, you'll go through thorough training in all aspects of pump use and intensive diabetes management. During this training you'll learn how to determine your insulin requirements, how to program your pump to safely administer the insulin and how to insert the catheter and care for the injection site.

Convenience and control

The main advantage of insulin pumps for many people is improved blood sugar control. The pump enables them to better match their insulin needs and insulin delivery. People who use insulin pumps are often able to achieve normal or near-normal blood sugar levels. Many people feel a pump also provides them a more flexible lifestyle.

Other advantages of an insulin pump include:

- Built-in safety alarms to let you know if the line's plugged, you're out of insulin or the battery is low
- Memory display of previous insulin delivery
- The ability to program multiple basal secretion rates to help prevent low blood sugar (hypoglycemia) and high blood sugar (hyperglycemia)

- The ability to gradually release insulin with meals, which is particularly useful if you're eating a high-fat meal because fat slows the absorption of carbohydrates and spreads out the production of glucose
- The ability to suspend or decrease insulin delivery during exercise and physical activity
- Quick release technology to easily disconnect the infusion tubing for situations such as showering, swimming or engaging in sexual activity
- Better blood sugar control in hard-to-control situations: travel, variable work shifts, erratic schedules

Who's a candidate?

Insulin pumps can be beneficial, but they aren't for everybody. If you're doing a good job of controlling your diabetes without a pump, the investment may not bring significant improvements in blood sugar control or your lifestyle.

To benefit from a pump you need to use it properly, monitor your blood sugar regularly and be willing to work closely with your doctor and diabetes educator. Some people find this regimen too demanding. The pumps also are expensive, costing up to $5,000. Many times, though, this cost is covered, at least in part, by insurance. Other drawbacks include risk of infection at the pump site, high blood sugar if the pump fails to deliver insulin and difficulty incorporating the pump into physical activities, such as swimming or contact sports.

Some women with diabetes who are pregnant or are contemplating pregnancy prefer an insulin pump. High blood sugar in early pregnancy can cause birth defects and illness in infants born to mothers with diabetes. Tight control of blood sugar reduces that risk. An insulin pump also may benefit people with:

Poor blood sugar control despite multiple injection therapy. An insulin pump uses only short-acting insulin. Frequent blood sugar monitoring helps determine your insulin needs.

Episodes of severe low blood sugar. A pump can reduce the incidence of severe hypoglycemia.

Extreme insulin sensitivity. A pump delivers fractional amounts of insulin at a time (0.05 to 0.10 unit increments), reducing the risk of hypoglycemia.

Problems of dawn phenomenon. Some people experience increased glucose production in the early morning hours and so need an increase in insulin. You can program your pump to increase insulin delivery during this time to counteract the rise in blood sugar.

Variable work or activity schedules. A pump allows you the freedom to program your insulin dosages to meet your changing needs.

Implantable insulin pumps

Researchers are experimenting with the possibility of implanting an insulin pump in your lower abdomen, making it more convenient and less noticeable. They're also working on new insulin preparations that can be used in implantable pumps, and they're studying ways to prevent buildup of insulin residue in the pump catheter, which could pose a problem. While some results are encouraging, much more work still needs to be done before implantable pumps will be ready for daily use.

Education is essential

For best results you need to know how your pump works and not be afraid of mechanical devices. It's essential that you have a clear understanding of the relationship between insulin, food and activity so that you can program your pump to help you out in changing situations. Even when using a pump, you still need to check your blood sugar four or more times a day.

Success also depends on whether you have realistic expectations. If you expect too much from your pump, you may be disappointed. It's only as good as the person controlling it. It's also important to meet regularly with people who have experience in pump use — your doctor, diabetes educator or dietitian — to make sure you're using the device correctly and all is going well.

Questions and answers

If I'm sick, especially if I'm vomiting, do I still take my usual doses of insulin?

Continue to take insulin, especially if you have type 1 diabetes, to prevent significant blood sugar elevations or accumulation of blood acids (ketoacidosis). Monitor your blood sugar frequently and adjust your insulin doses as necessary. Keep well hydrated by drinking fluids that contain calories. If your blood sugar is persistently above 300 mg/dL or you're unable to keep fluids down because of vomiting, call your doctor.

If I'm scheduled for surgery, do I take my insulin as usual?

Before surgery you'll be fasting. If you're injecting insulin, omit the short-acting doses. The general rule of thumb is to take half of your usual intermediate-acting dose, but verify this with your doctor. If you're using a pump, keep the basal insulin dose going. Remember to check your blood sugar frequently prior to and following unique circumstances such as surgery.

What should I do if I forget to give myself an insulin injection?

If you miss just one dose, it's generally not a problem. Wait until the next scheduled time for an injection and give yourself the regular amount. Don't double it to make up for the missed injection.

I've heard researchers are working on alternative ways to deliver insulin. What's the status of this research?

Insulin research continues on many fronts, including less invasive methods of delivery. Scientists are experimenting with two types of inhaled insulin preparations. One is delivered through your mouth and the other through your nose. Much work still needs to be done, though, before researchers can evaluate whether these methods would be effective and reliable.

Chapter 8

Medications for type 2 diabetes

U nlike type 1 diabetes, which requires daily insulin, treatment of type 2 disease is more complex because you can take several routes to manage your blood sugar (glucose). For many people with type 2 diabetes, lifestyle changes alone can control it. For others, these changes aren't enough. Sooner or later, most people need the help of medication.

A variety of drug options exist for treatment of type 2 diabetes. In addition to insulin, five categories of oral medications are available. Each of these classes of medications has a different chemical structure and its own method for lowering blood sugar. Some oral diabetes medications stimulate your pancreas to produce more insulin, others help your body reduce its resistance to insulin, and still others slow your body's absorption of carbohydrates.

To effectively control your blood sugar, you may need more than one drug. Oral medications can be taken in combination with each other or in combination with insulin. Your doctor will determine if you need medication to control your blood sugar and which type. Most people begin with an oral drug.

Sulfonylureas

Sulfonylureas (SUL-fuh-nil-uh-REE-uhs) have been used for decades to control blood sugar. The drugs work by stimulating beta cells in your pancreas to produce more insulin. So, to benefit from the medication, your pancreas must be able to produce some insulin on its own.

Sulfonylureas include the following medications:

- Chlorpropamide (Diabinese)
- Glimepiride (Amaryl)
- Glipizide (Glucotrol, Glucotrol XL)
- Glyburide (DiaBeta, Glynase PresTab, Micronase)
- Tolazamide (Tolinase, Ronase)
- Tolbutamide (Orinase)

Glipizide, glyburide and glimepiride — second-generation sulfonylureas — are the most commonly used sulfonylureas. These newer versions of the original drugs are less likely to cause low blood sugar (hypoglycemia), and they don't linger as long in your circulatory system, reducing your risk of complications from medication use. Glipizide is available in two forms: a short-acting version and a sustained-release (XL) version. With the sustained-release version, you take the medication less often.

An advantage of the drug glimepiride is that it's safer for individuals with impaired kidney function because the condition doesn't affect the absorption and action of the drug. With other sulfonylureas, impaired kidney function causes the drugs to accumulate, increasing your risk of low blood sugar.

Possible side effects

Low blood sugar is the most common side effect of sulfonylureas, especially during the first 4 months of therapy when the decrease in your fasting blood sugar is the most dramatic. You're at a much greater risk of developing hypoglycemia if you have impaired liver or kidney (renal) function. In fact, these conditions may influence your doctor not to prescribe a sulfonylurea. Research also suggests sulfonylureas may increase your risk of heart problems. However, one large study (United Kingdom Prospective Diabetes Study) found that people taking sulfonylureas didn't appear to have an increased risk of heart problems.

Precautions

Doing anything that reduces your blood sugar after you've taken a sulfonylurea, such as skipping a meal or exercising more than usual, can lead to low blood sugar. Taking alcohol or certain drugs with sulfonylureas, including decongestants, also can cause low blood sugar by boosting the effects of the medication. Medications such as steroids, beta blockers, niacin and the acne drug Retin-A can decrease the effectiveness of sulfonylureas.

Talk with your doctor before taking any over-the-counter or prescription medication. It's also best to have all of your prescriptions filled at the same pharmacy so that your pharmacist can be alert to any potential drug interactions.

Meglitinides

Meglitinides (muh-GLIT-in-ides) are chemically different than sulfonylureas, but their effects are similar. These medications cause a rapid, but short-lived release of insulin by your pancreas. Because they work quickly and their effects diminish rapidly, the medications are taken with meals, kicking into action shortly thereafter, when your blood sugar level is highest.

Repaglinide (Prandin) is the only drug in this class to receive Food and Drug Administration (FDA) approval. Other drugs are being developed and are expected to be available in the near future.

Possible side effects

Like sulfonylureas, meglitinides can cause low blood sugar. However, they stimulate insulin production only if your blood sugar level is high, so the risk of hypoglycemia is lower.

Precautions

Similar to sulfonylureas, be aware of possible drug interactions if you're taking other medications or using alcohol.

Biguanides

Biguanides (by-GWAN-ides) improve your body's response to insulin, decreasing insulin resistance. Between meals your liver releases stored sugar into your bloodstream. Among people with type 2 diabetes, this process is frequently exaggerated. Biguanides reduce the amount of sugar your liver releases during fasting. As a result, you need less insulin to transport sugar from your blood to your individual cells.

Metformin (Glucophage) is the only drug in this class available in the United States. An important benefit of the medication is that it's associated with less weight gain than other diabetes medications. For this reason, it's often prescribed to people with type 2 diabetes who are overweight. In addition, the drug may slightly reduce blood fats — cholesterol and triglycerides — which tend to be higher than normal in people with type 2 diabetes. Metformin also is available in extended release tablets (Glucophage XR).

Possible side effects

Metformin is generally quite tolerable, but it can produce side effects in some people. Let your doctor know if you experience any of the following:

- Changes in taste, such as an unpleasant metallic taste in your mouth
- Loss of appetite
- Nausea or vomiting
- Abdominal bloating, discomfort or pain
- Gas or diarrhea
- Skin rash

These effects usually occur during the first few weeks of taking the medication and decrease with time. They're less likely to occur if you take the medication with food and if you start out at a low dosage and gradually increase the amount you take.

When combined with another diabetes medication, such as a sulfonylurea, a meglitinide or insulin, metformin may cause low blood sugar. A rare but serious side effect of metformin is lactic acidosis, a buildup of lactic acid in your body that can result from excessive accumulation of the drug. You're more likely to experience this condition if you have kidney disease, congestive heart failure or any other disease that may cause your body to produce too much lactic acid. Symptoms of lactic acidosis include:

- Tiredness
- Weakness
- Muscle aches
- Breathing difficulties
- Abdominal pain
- Dizziness
- Drowsiness

Precautions

Metformin and alcohol don't mix well. If you drink alcohol daily or you occasionally overindulge, metformin can produce lactic acidosis, making you sick. If your doctor recommends metformin and you drink alcohol, mention your use of alcohol to your doctor.

If you take the gastrointestinal medication cimetidine (Tagamet), your dose of metformin may need to be lowered because of a possible drug interaction. Cimetidine can interfere with your kidney's ability to rid your body of metformin, causing a buildup of the drug and possible lactic acidosis. Because of potential for lactic acidosis, it's also important that you stop taking metformin prior to undergoing any procedure involving the use of an intravenous (IV) dye. IV dyes are sometimes used in imaging procedures, such as a computed tomography (CT) scan.

Alpha-glucosidase inhibitors

Alpha-glucosidase (gloo-KOE-sih-days) inhibitors block the action of enzymes in the digestive tract that break down carbohydrates into sugar, delaying the digestion of carbohydrates. Sugar is absorbed into your bloodstream more slowly than usual, limiting the rapid rise in blood sugar that usually occurs right after a meal.

Two medications are in this class: acarbose (Precose) and miglitol (Glyset). You take them with each meal. Because the drugs aren't as effective as sulfonylureas or metformin in controlling fasting sugar levels, they're typically prescribed if your blood sugar reaches its highest levels right after meals (postprandial elevations).

Possible side effects

Alpha-glucosidase inhibitors are quite safe and effective. But they cause gastrointestinal side effects that can be bothersome, including abdominal bloating or discomfort, gas or diarrhea. These effects usually occur during the first few weeks of taking the medication and decrease with time. If you start with a low dose of the medication and gradually increase the amount you take, you're more likely to experience only mild instead of severe symptoms.

When taken with another oral diabetes medication, such as a sulfonylurea or insulin, you run an increased risk of experiencing low blood sugar. If you do experience hypoglycemia, drink milk or use glucose tablets or gel to treat it. Don't use table sugar or fruit juice because alpha-glucosidase inhibitors block the absorption of these sugars.

Precautions

Because of possible digestive side effects, you shouldn't take acarbose or miglitol if you have the following medical conditions:

- Irritable bowel syndrome
- Ulcerative colitis or Crohn's disease
- Partial intestinal obstruction or a predisposition for this problem
- A chronic malabsorption disorder, such as celiac disease

If taken in high doses, acarbose and miglitol can injure your liver. Fortunately, the damage is usually reversible by reducing the dosage of the medication or discontinuing it.

Thiazolidinediones

Most people with type 2 diabetes have a resistance to insulin that prevents the hormone from working properly. Thiazolidinediones (THIGH-ah-ZOL-ih-deen-DYE-owns) help reduce blood sugar by making your body tissues more sensitive to insulin. The more effective insulin is at escorting sugar from your blood into your cells, the less sugar that remains in your bloodstream. Thiazolidinediones also keep your liver from overproducing glucose. Another common benefit of thiazolidinediones is a decrease in triglycerides.

This class of medications includes the drugs pioglitazone (Actos) and rosiglitazone (Avandia). It also included the medication troglitazone (Rezulin), which has been withdrawn from the market.

Possible side effects

Side effects from the medications may include swelling, weight gain and fatigue. A rare but serious side effect of thiazolidinediones is liver injury. Before you take pioglitazone or rosiglitazone, your doctor should have you undergo blood tests to assess the health of your liver. It's also important to have your liver checked every 2

The removal of Rezulin

The first thiazolidinedione to be approved by the Food and Drug Administration (FDA) was taken off the market only a couple of years later. Troglitazone (Rezulin) was approved in 1997 with high expectations of helping people with type 2 diabetes who didn't benefit from other oral medications. However, shortly after the drug became available, cases of liver failure began to appear. In March 2000 the FDA asked the manufacturer of troglitazone to remove the product from the market.

Risk of liver damage from other drugs in this class of medications, rosiglitazone (Avandia) and pioglitazone (Actos), appears to be lower because they're handled (metabolized) differently by your body. The FDA does, however, require that the medications carry warnings regarding the potential for liver damage, and it recommends that people taking rosiglitazone and pioglitazone have periodic blood tests to assess their liver health.

months during the first year of therapy. Contact your doctor right away if you experience any signs and symptoms of liver damage:

- Nausea and vomiting
- Abdominal pain
- Fatigue
- Loss of appetite
- Dark urine
- Yellowing of your skin (jaundice)

Precautions

Thiazolidinediones are generally best absorbed if you take them with a meal. Taken alone, the medications don't cause low blood sugar, but when used with a sulfonylurea or insulin, hypoglycemia can occur. If you're taking birth control pills, thiazolidinediones may make the contraceptives less effective.

Insulin

Insulin is generally associated with treatment of type 1 diabetes, but it's also an effective medication for treating type 2 diabetes. You may take insulin alone or you may use it in combination with an oral diabetes medication.

Your doctor may recommend insulin injections if you have poor control of your diabetes, either because your pancreas isn't making enough insulin or you aren't responding to other medications. Your doctor also may turn first to insulin if:

- Your fasting blood sugar level is markedly high — more than 300 milligrams of glucose per deciliter of blood (mg/dL) — and you have a high level of ketones in your urine (see Chapter 2 for more information on ketones).

- You have a markedly high fasting blood sugar level and are experiencing symptoms of diabetes.

- You have gestational diabetes that can't be controlled.

You may need to take insulin for a short period to help bring your diabetes under control, or you may use the medication long-term to maintain your blood sugar within a safe range. Short-term insulin use also may prompt long-lasting improvements in your metabolism, as well as allow beta cells in your pancreas time to recover. These cells can be damaged when exposed to high levels of sugar. For more information on insulin, see Chapter 7.

Drug combinations

The goal of combination therapy is to maximize the glucose-lowering effects of diabetes medications. By combining medications from different drug classes, the medications may work in two different ways to control your blood sugar. The most common combination therapy is to take two separate drugs at the same time. Two drugs also may be combined into one pill (see "A combination pill," on page 128).

Some doctors prescribe three drugs at a time. More studies are necessary to determine the benefits of triple-drug therapy, but this may be an option if a combination of two oral medications doesn't achieve your goal. Each class of oral medication can be combined with one another.

A sulfonylurea and metformin

Sulfonylureas are often the base of combination therapy because of their ability to boost and maintain insulin secretion. A sulfonylurea combined with metformin is the most extensively studied drug combination. The medications seem to work more effectively together than they do individually, reducing fasting blood sugar by up to 70 mg/dL and glycated hemoglobin by up to 2 percent. Metformin also is beneficial in that it can help people who are overweight avoid additional weight gain, and in some cases, lose weight. Common side effects of this drug combination include nausea, diarrhea and a risk of low blood sugar.

A sulfonylurea and an alpha-glucosidase inhibitor
Combining acarbose or miglitol with a sulfonylurea is especially effective if you experience significant spikes in your blood sugar immediately following meals. Possible side effects include abdominal cramping, gas and diarrhea. You also may experience low blood sugar. Again, be sure to treat episodes of hypoglycemia with milk or glucose tablets or gel because alpha-glucosidase inhibitors block the absorption of table sugar and fruit juice.

A sulfonylurea and a thiazolidinedione
This is one of the newest approaches in combination therapy. Adding a thiazolidinedione medication to a sulfonylurea makes sense when the maximum dose of a sulfonylurea isn't working for you, you're overweight and your cells are highly insulin resistant. This combination also increases your risk of low blood sugar because thiazolidinediones improve your body's use of insulin stimulated by sulfonylureas.

Metformin and an alpha-glucosidase inhibitor
Studies consistently show that the combination of acarbose (an alpha-glucosidase inhibitor) and metformin is more effective in reducing blood sugar following meals than metformin alone. Because miglitol (another alpha-glucosidase inhibitor) is a newer medication, it hasn't been studied in combination with metformin as often as acarbose has been, but the same benefits are likely to apply. Possible side effects from combining metformin and an alpha-glucosidase inhibitor are the same as those associated with using metformin or an alpha-glucosidase inhibitor alone. Gastrointestinal symptoms are the most common side effect.

Metformin and a thiazolidinedione

The FDA has approved the thiazolidinediones rosiglitazone and pioglitazone for use with metformin. The combination therapy is more effective at reducing blood sugar than either class of medication alone. The precautions and side effects are the same as those listed for these drugs individually.

Oral medications and insulin

Combining insulin with an oral medication can help both drugs work more effectively. The combination also can lower your daily insulin requirements and may limit weight gain associated with insulin therapy alone.

A sulfonylurea and insulin. Years ago, if you couldn't control your blood sugar with a sulfonylurea, your doctor would likely take you off the oral drug and prescribe insulin alone. Studies now show that adding a dose of insulin at bedtime to your regular dosage of a sulfonylurea may improve blood sugar control.

At first glance, a sulfonylurea and insulin don't appear to be a likely combination because they both boost insulin levels. However, they promote the circulation of insulin in different parts of your body. Using a sulfonylurea with insulin may allow you to use lower doses of insulin and achieve the same control. This treatment regimen is called BIDS (bedtime insulin daytime sulfonylurea) therapy. BIDS therapy also may be useful if a combination of a sulfonylurea and metformin hasn't worked for you.

A combination pill

Most combination therapies involve taking two separate drugs. Recently, the Food and Drug Administration approved the first combination pill. It contains the medications glyburide and metformin in one pill. Called Glucovance, the medication may be used alone or in combination with additional glyburide or metformin, or a sulfonylurea.

The most common side effects of Glucovance are diarrhea and nausea. In rare cases, it may lead to lactic acidosis.

Metformin and insulin. Similar to a sulfonylurea combination, combining metformin with insulin can reduce your insulin dose. Metformin helps your liver become more sensitive to insulin, making better use of it. Metformin also counteracts the problem of weight gain associated with insulin use. In fact, you may actually lose weight when using this combination. One theory is that metformin reduces appetite, causing you to consume fewer calories.

An alpha-glucosidase inhibitor and insulin. The FDA has approved the combination of acarbose (an alpha-glucosidase inhibitor) and insulin. The newer alpha-glucosidase inhibitor miglitol hasn't been extensively studied in combination with insulin. Acarbose delays the absorption of carbohydrates, reducing your daily need for insulin. Because acarbose slows carbohydrate absorption, it also increases risk of low blood sugar that can occur with insulin therapy.

A thiazolidinedione and insulin. This pairing is the most-studied of the insulin combination therapies. If your blood sugar is well controlled, taking a thiazolidinedione with insulin can reduce the amount of insulin you need each day. If you have trouble controlling your blood sugar, adding a thiazolidinedione may help you better regulate your blood sugar levels. A side effect of this combination is low blood sugar, along with the previously mentioned side effects of thiazolidinediones.

New diabetes drugs

Several new diabetes medications are being developed and studied. Two treatments likely to be approved in the near future are glucagon-like peptide (GLP-1) and pramlintide acetate (Symlin).

Glucagon-like peptide (GLP-1)

The hormone GLP-1 lowers blood sugar levels by increasing insulin production and decreasing sugar secretion by your liver. It appears to work best if your pancreas secretes at least some insulin. The downfall of the drug is that it can't be taken orally because it's metabolized so quickly. The only way for GLP-1 to be effective is for it to be delivered via an injection or insulin pump.

Pramlintide acetate

Pramlintide acetate (Symlin) is a synthetic replica (analog) of the human beta cell hormone amylin. Beta cells are found in your pancreas and are critical to insulin production. Studies show that adding Symlin to insulin therapy improves blood sugar control without significant side effects or risk of low blood sugar.

Questions and answers

What should I do if I forget to take my medication?

If you're 6 or more hours late with your medication, don't take it, and don't double the next dose. Continue to follow your regular medication schedule.

Can I use an insulin pump if I have type 2 diabetes?

A pump is an option if you take insulin, no matter if you have type 1 or type 2 diabetes. Most people with type 2 diabetes don't need a pump because they do well with less intensive treatment. However, with proper documentation, Medicare may cover the expense of a pump if you have type 2 diabetes. For more information on insulin pumps, see Chapter 7.

Will any herbal remedies help treat type 2 diabetes?

Some people with diabetes do take herbal remedies in an effort to ease their symptoms, even though the effectiveness and side effects of these remedies are generally unknown. The American Diabetes Association cautions against their use because little research exists to prove the remedies are safe and effective.

A limited study of the herb ginseng conducted by researchers at the University of Toronto shows that it may be helpful in reducing blood sugar after meals. Ginseng is thought to delay digestion and possibly the absorption of carbohydrates. More research is under way to investigate possible benefits of the herb and whether it produces side effects.

Chapter 9

Transplantation

T he last few decades have shown that medication and lifestyle changes can effectively control diabetes, but a common question lingers: What about a cure?

Presently, there is no cure for diabetes. Researchers continue to explore treatment therapies that they hope could one day bring about a cure. One area of study that continues to receive a lot of attention is transplantation. Since the late 1970s, doctors have performed pancreas transplants to halt or reverse complications of diabetes, and the procedure has met with some success. But the treatment method gaining the most attention these days is a procedure called islet cell transplantation. Researchers have known for some time that transplanting the cells that produce insulin (islet cells) may provide a possible cure for type 1 diabetes. The process has been ridden with obstacles, but there's some evidence researchers may be getting closer to their goal.

Pancreas transplantation

In 1966 doctors first transplanted a pancreas in a human being with type 1 diabetes. More surgeries followed but the survival rate among people receiving a new pancreas was so low that limited transplants occurred. By 1978 improved medications, new surgical techniques and the selection of healthier patients brought better results. To date, surgeons have performed well over 10,000 pancreas transplants. In the United States, more than 900 pancreas transplants occur annually.

Most pancreas transplants are either done in conjunction with or following a kidney transplant. Kidney failure is one of the most common complications of diabetes. Your kidneys perform a number of crucial functions, including filtering wastes from your blood and controlling your body's fluid and chemical balance. A kidney transplant can restore your body's ability to perform these essential tasks. Receiving a new pancreas at the same time doesn't jeopardize, and may actually improve, kidney survival. In addition, a new pancreas can restore your blood sugar (glucose) levels to normal.

After a successful pancreas transplantation, many people with diabetes don't need to use insulin anymore or take frequent blood sugar measurements. They're also no longer at risk of soaring or dropping blood sugar levels and the dangers they bring. On the flip side, pancreas transplants aren't always successful. Besides the risk inherent in any major surgery, your body can reject the new organ days or years after the transplant. Your immune system treats the new organ as a foreign invader and tries to reject (destroy) it. Because of this, you'll likely need to take immunosuppressive drugs the rest of your life. These drugs prevent your immune system from reacting in this manner.

The only time a pancreas transplant is performed alone — without a prior or simultaneous kidney transplant — is if your kidneys are still relatively healthy but your diabetes isn't responding to conventional treatment. Pancreas-only transplants are less common.

Unlike kidney transplants, in which a living person may donate a kidney, most pancreases used for transplantation come from people who have just died.

Are you a candidate?
Candidates for pancreas transplants generally have type 1 diabetes, are age 45 or younger and don't have other health conditions that would place them at high risk of complications from major surgery.

There are three groups of candidates:

Group 1. People in this group are candidates for a combined kidney and pancreas transplant. They have kidney failure from diabetes but are otherwise in acceptable health. Most people who receive a donor pancreas fall into this group.

Group 2. People in this group have already received a kidney transplant and now are in need of a pancreas transplant to control their diabetes.

Group 3. People in this group have diabetes and aren't experiencing kidney problems, but they could benefit from a pancreas transplant to control their diabetes, in hopes of preventing complications. You might fall into this category if you experience frequent and severe bouts of high blood sugar (hyperglycemia) or low blood sugar (hypoglycemia) that require medical attention. You might also be a candidate if insulin therapy isn't successfully controlling your blood sugar.

Success rates

Group 1 has the highest success rate from pancreas transplantation. Approximately 85 percent of people who receive a combination kidney and pancreas transplant no longer require insulin a year after surgery. Among people in groups 2 and 3, 70 percent and 60 percent, respectively, are off insulin a year after the transplant. As more effective immunosuppressive drugs are developed, success rates are expected to improve.

There are many possible reasons why a combination kidney and pancreas transplant has a higher success rate. One reason is that the pancreas induces a much stronger immune response than a kidney. Therefore a pancreas transplant alone often requires larger doses of immunosuppressive drugs, including steroids, that can jeopardize kidney function and the transplanted pancreas.

Risk of rejection

Rejection of your new pancreas is one of the greatest risks of pancreas transplant surgery. Rejection occurs when your immune system identifies a new organ as a foreign invader and attacks it, just as it does a foreign virus or bacteria. Risk of organ rejection with a pancreas transplant is much higher — either alone or in combination with a kidney — than with a kidney transplant.

New drugs that suppress your immune system are making it easier for doctors to control incidents of rejection. The downside of immunosuppressive drugs is their high cost and their potential side effects, including a higher risk of infection and organ injury.

For these reasons, transplantation generally isn't an option if you're in good control of your diabetes and you aren't experiencing significant complications. The side effects of immunosuppressive drugs could be more dangerous to your overall health than your diabetes itself.

Making a decision

Many factors must be considered when deciding if you should have a pancreas transplant. The stage and progression of your kidney disease, as well as the cost of the procedure, are among the issues you should discuss with an experienced transplant team. If your diabetes is causing serious complications, the best choice may be to wait for a combined kidney and pancreas transplant. A combined transplant is generally the most efficient and cost-effective option.

If your diabetes is generally under control and your main concern is to avoid dialysis, then a kidney transplant from a living donor may be the best choice. Living donor kidney transplants have a slightly higher rate of success than a transplant using a donor kidney from an individual who has just died. If necessary, a pancreas transplant could still be possible later on to control worsening diabetes.

Transplants come with a hefty price tag. Hospitalization and doctor fees can run up to $100,000, and immunosuppressive drugs can cost anywhere from $5,000 to $20,000 a year, depending on your individual needs. Medicare and many insurance plans generally cover kidney and combined kidney-pancreas transplants, but not pancreas transplants alone. That's because, to date, they haven't been found to be as successful in the long term.

Islet cell transplantation

For decades researchers and surgeons have regarded islet cells as a possible key to a diabetes cure. A human pancreas contains about 1 million islets. These cells make up about 2 percent of the pancreas. Beta cells, the cells that produce insulin, make up 75 percent to 80 percent of the islets. The remainder of pancreatic cells produce enzymes to help digest food. In people with type 1 diabetes, their immune system attacks and destroys islet cells, so their pancreas is no longer able to produce insulin.

Researchers have looked at different methods of producing new islet cells. One such method is transplantation of individual cells. Doctors extract islet cells from the pancreas of a person who has just died and then infuse them via a catheter into the liver of the person with diabetes. The cells spread throughout the liver, establish new vascular attachments and begin to produce insulin.

Your liver instead of your pancreas is the location for the transplant because:

- It's easier and less invasive to access the large vein (portal vein) in your liver than a pancreatic vein.
- Islet cells that grow in the liver still closely mimic normal insulin secretion.

For years this procedure has been fraught with problems. The cells are very fragile, and the transplant process is difficult. In addition, immunosuppressive drugs given to prevent cell rejection often worsened the recipient's diabetes. However, recent studies are instilling a renewed sense of hope. Improved surgical techniques and new immunosuppresive medications are producing more successful outcomes.

A comeback

In 1999, scientists in Canada transplanted islet cells into eight people seriously ill with type 1 diabetes. They used a new combination of immunosuppressive drugs that doesn't include steroids, which are toxic to your insulin-producing cells. They also used fresh islet cells instead of frozen cells, as has been the usual practice. In addition, the researchers increased the number of islet cells they infused into the recipients, improving the odds of an adequate number of cells surviving the transplant process.

Results of the transplants, published a year later, found that all eight people no longer required insulin injections. They haven't rejected the transplanted cells nor have their immune systems attacked the new cells, as they did their original islet cells. Canadian researchers attribute this success to the use of fresh islet cells and improved immunosuppressive drugs.

Current status

One of the main advantages of islet cell transplantation is that it's less invasive than pancreas transplantation. The procedure takes just a short while and the individual remains fully conscious while the islet cells are being transplanted. Islet cell transplantation also isn't as costly as pancreas transplantation. Because it's still considered experimental, however, the procedure isn't covered by medical insurance.

One of the biggest obstacles facing the procedure is the availability of fresh islet cells. There's a shortage of organ donors in the United States, and the supply of islet cells isn't reliable. Another challenge is the ability to isolate the cells.

Scientists from California are experimenting with a procedure to grow human beta cells in a laboratory. The research is still in its early stages and contains difficulties of its own. Among other things, the same properties that allow for growth and reproduction of the insulin-producing cells may cause cancer. The researchers have developed techniques they believe negate cancer potential, but they're still looking for risk of tumor formation.

Meanwhile, additional studies are under way to learn more about the long-term effects of islet cell transplantation and to try to duplicate the success of the Canadian study. Researchers hope to know in 1 to 2 years if the immediate effects of the procedure are long lasting. There's also the uncertainty of complications from the newer immunosuppressive medications.

Questions and answers

Is pancreas or islet cell transplantation only an option for people with type 1 diabetes? Can people with type 2 disease benefit too?
Most studies to date have involved individuals with type 1 diabetes. With improved techniques and outcomes, it's possible these therapies could one day be available to people with type 2 disease. But transplantation may not improve type 2 diabetes, especially if your individual cells have a severe resistance to insulin.

Can islet cells be transplanted into a child with newly diagnosed type 1 diabetes?
That's the long-term goal of researchers: To catch the disease early and eliminate it before it has a chance to do any damage. Until recently, islet cell transplantation would never have been considered for a child, let alone most adults, with type 1 diabetes. This thinking could possibly change if current research efforts are successful. Presently, though, only people with type 1 diabetes who are very ill are being considered for transplants.

Are there any studies looking at ways to eliminate the need for the lifelong use of immunosuppressive drugs following a transplant?
Yes. A number of research centers throughout the world are investigating tolergenic drugs. These newer and less potent medications can trick your body into accepting the transplanted cells and organs. The drugs work by shutting off a small part of your immune system — just enough to keep the new cells from being attacked. If the medications work, you would no longer need to take immunosuppressive drugs indefinitely.

How do I get on a donor organ recipient list?
You and your doctor need to determine if transplantation is the proper treatment for you. If you decide that a transplant is the best choice, you'll need to be evaluated by an experienced transplant team before being placed on an organ recipient list.

How do I find out more about participating in clinical trials for islet cell transplantation?

Talk with your doctor to see if he or she thinks you would be an appropriate candidate. You also can contact the American Diabetes Association (ADA) to learn more about islet cell transplantation research and its progress. The ADA's address, phone number and Web site address are listed on page 185.

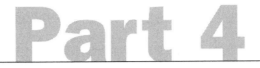

Part 4

Living Well

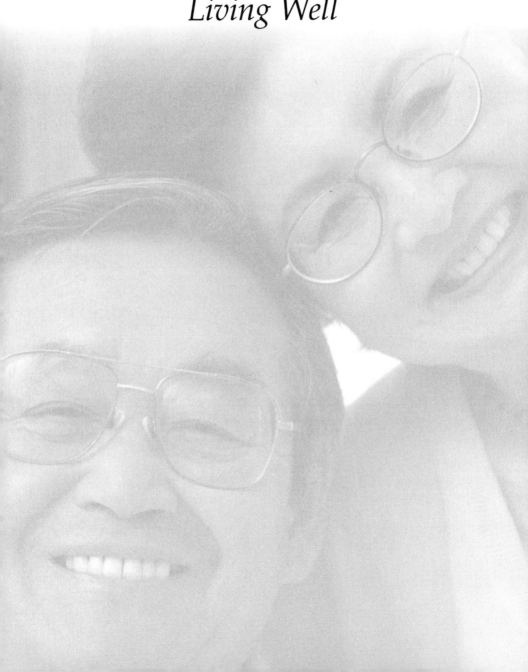

Chapter 10

Important tests: Are you getting them?

A few weeks to months following your diagnosis, managing your diabetes should start to become routine. You'll gradually develop a pattern for testing your blood sugar (glucose), exercising and eating. But you often may wonder, "How am I doing?" You'd like to know if your daily efforts at controlling your blood sugar are paying off and keeping other health problems at bay.

You can find the answer you're looking for by keeping in regular contact with your health care team and making sure you receive appropriate tests during your checkups. These tests can evaluate how well you're doing in controlling your blood sugar and spot potential problems.

Regular checkups are important because they:

- Provide your doctor an opportunity to check for early stages of diabetes complications. Many potential complications show up early in simple blood and urine tests and examinations performed in your doctor's office.

- Allow you and your doctor to review your successes and difficulties at meeting your blood sugar goals.

- Give you an opportunity to hear suggestions from members of your health care team on how to meet your goals.

Assembling your team

Successful management of diabetes often involves working with more than one individual. Your health care team may include the following professionals:

A doctor. Your primary doctor may be a diabetes specialist (endocrinologist) or a primary care physician.

A physician extender. A physician extender works closely with your doctor and may assist with your care. This person may be a physician's assistant or a nurse practitioner.

A diabetes educator. A diabetes educator is certified in teaching people with diabetes how to manage their disease. This person is often a registered nurse.

A registered dietitian. A registered dietitian works with you to develop a healthy eating plan to help control your blood sugar levels.

How often you should see your doctor or other members of your health care team depends on what's happening with your health. If you're having trouble keeping your blood sugar levels down or if you're changing medication, you may need to contact a member of your health care team weekly. Your doctor may even recommend that you stop in as often as once a day until your blood sugar and insulin levels stabilize.

In general, though, if you're feeling good and keeping your blood sugar within the range that you and your doctor have agreed upon, you probably won't need to see your doctor more than four times a year — once every 3 months. If you reach and are able to maintain your blood sugar goals, the visits may be even further apart.

What to expect during a checkup

Your doctor will likely begin your examination by asking you questions about your blood sugar readings and overall health: How have you been feeling? Have you been experiencing any new symptoms or problems? Have you been able to keep your blood sugar within your target range? It's important to bring your daily log of blood sugar readings with you to your appointment so your doctor can review it. He or she will be especially concerned about any episodes of high or low blood sugar, and what caused them.

Other issues your doctor may want to cover include:

- Temporary adjustments you made to your treatment program, including changes in medication, to accommodate for high or low blood sugar readings

- Problems you're having in following your treatment program

- Emotional and social problems you may be experiencing

- Changes in your use of tobacco or alcohol

During your checkup a member of your health care team will also:

Check your blood pressure. Like diabetes, high blood pressure (hypertension) can damage your blood vessels. Diabetes and high blood pressure are frequently associated, and when teamed together they can speed you in the direction of a heart attack or stroke. If your blood pressure is high, you may need to take medication to control it. Controlling your high blood pressure can help prevent diabetes complications.

Check your weight. If you have diabetes and you're overweight, losing weight can help you control your blood sugar. If you take a diabetes medication, weight loss may reduce your need for medication. Gaining weight can make it more difficult for you to manage high blood sugar.

Check your feet. At each visit your doctor should do a brief examination of your feet. At least once a year he or she should perform a thorough foot examination. During a thorough exam, your doctor is looking for:

- Breaks in the skin, which could lead to an infection

- Foot pulses, which indicate if you have good blood circulation in the foot, and a sense of touch, which indicates if sensory nerves in the foot are working properly

- Normal range of motion, to make sure there is no muscle or bone damage

- Bony deformations or evidence of increased pressure, such as calluses, which may suggest you need different shoes

If a problem is identified, you'll need to examine your feet regularly to make sure the condition doesn't worsen. If you're unable to examine your feet yourself, recruit the help of a family member or a close friend.

Request blood and urine tests. Simple blood and urine tests can detect early signs of diabetes complications, such as kidney disease. The earlier you discover and treat emerging problems, the better your chances of stopping, or at least slowing, the damage.

The following four tests are especially important. Three of them examine your blood and one examines your urine.

Glycated hemoglobin test

A glycated hemoglobin test is the most effective tool for determining how well you're managing your blood sugar. This blood test is different from a fasting blood sugar test or a daily finger prick, both of which only measure your blood sugar at any given moment. A glycated hemoglobin test — also known as the hemoglobin A-1C test — indicates how well you've controlled your blood sugar during the past 2 to 3 months.

How does it work?

Your red blood cells contain hemoglobin, a protein that gives blood its red color and that carries oxygen from your lungs to all the cells in your body. When a red blood cell is first formed, it has no sugar attached to it. But as the cell is exposed to sugar in your blood, some of the sugar may attach itself to hemoglobin in the cell. This is known as glycated or glycosylated hemoglobin, terms from an ancient Greek work that means "sweet." How much hemoglobin may become glycated depends on the average amount of sugar in your bloodstream.

Normally, a small percentage of your hemoglobin has sugar attached to it. If you have diabetes and keep your blood sugar within a normal or near-normal range, your glycated hemoglobin value will reflect this by being similar to that of an individual without diabetes. If you've had trouble controlling your blood sugar during the past couple of months, the test will indicate a higher percentage of glycated hemoglobin.

To check your glycated hemoglobin level, blood is drawn from a vein in your arm and examined in a laboratory. The normal range for glycated hemoglobin values varies among laboratories across the country. It's important that this variation be taken into consideration when your doctor or other health team member interprets the results of your test.

How often should I have it done?

If you use insulin to control your diabetes — whether you have type 1 or type 2 — your doctor will probably suggest that you have a glycated hemoglobin test four times a year. If you have type 2 diabetes and are able to control your blood sugar levels with diet and exercise or oral medications, you may not need the test that often.

How does it help?

A glycated hemoglobin test can be beneficial in many ways. Say for instance you've been having trouble maintaining a normal blood sugar level and your doctor is debating whether to prescribe medication or a more aggressive exercise plan. Your doctor may have you increase the amount of time you exercise for 2 or 3 months and then come in for a glycated hemoglobin test. If the test produces a normal reading, your doctor knows that increased exercise may be all that you need to control your blood sugar, and you may not have to take medication.

Results of the glycated hemoglobin test also indicate your risk of diabetic complications. The higher the reading, the greater your risk of developing other health problems.

For people in control of their blood sugar, the test is confirmation that they should continue to follow the steps they're taking. In addition, the test is a way to alert you and your doctor to potential problems. If you've had normal glycated hemoglobin readings for several months or years and suddenly you have an abnormal reading, that may be a sign that you need to make modifications to your treatment plan, including more frequent blood sugar testing.

Lipids test

This blood test measures the level of fats (lipids) in your blood. After you eat, your body digests the fat in your food and releases it into your bloodstream in two forms, cholesterol and triglycerides.

For the test, blood is drawn from a vein in your arm and sent to a laboratory where blood fats are measured. To get an accurate reading, it's best to fast for at least 12 hours before blood is drawn.

Cholesterol

Cholesterol is a waxy, fatlike substance. Your body needs cholesterol for making cell walls and insulating your nerves. Your liver also uses it to make bile acids, which help digest your food. It's when you have too much cholesterol — especially too much of a certain kind — that trouble may occur.

People with type 2 diabetes often have unhealthy levels of cholesterol. That's partly because most people with type 2 diabetes are overweight and excess weight contributes to higher cholesterol and triglyceride levels. Genetic factors also can produce unhealthy cholesterol levels.

Cholesterol can't travel through your bloodstream in its original form. During digestion your body coats cholesterol with protein. Once coated, the package is called a lipoprotein (lip-oe-PRO-teen), or a fat-filled protein. Cholesterol is packaged in three forms:

Low-density lipoprotein (LDL). This form is often described as "bad" cholesterol. One way to remember this is to think of the first L as meaning "lousy." If you have too much LDL cholesterol in your blood, your body's cells become saturated with cholesterol, and the cholesterol is deposited on your artery walls, where it accumulates and hardens. This hard substance, called plaque, begins to narrow and harden artery walls, making it more difficult for blood to pass through them. If the flow of blood to your heart is severely diminished or completely interrupted, you'll have a heart attack. If blood flow to part of your brain is blocked, you'll have a stroke.

In people with diabetes, LDL cholesterol molecules tend to be smaller and more dense than in people without diabetes. The more dense the molecules, the more damage they can do.

High-density lipoprotein (HDL). Unlike LDL cholesterol, which contains mostly cholesterol, HDL cholesterol contains mostly protein. This form of cholesterol is often described as the "good" cholesterol. Think of the H as standing for "healthy." HDL cholesterol actually picks up cholesterol deposited on your artery walls and transports it to your liver for disposal.

Very-low-density lipoprotein (VLDL). Very-low-density lipoprotein is mainly composed of triglycerides, along with smaller amounts of cholesterol and protein. Elevations in VLDL cholesterol also can increase your risk of heart disease.

Triglycerides

Triglycerides are the chemicals in which most fat exists in your body. Your body converts calories it doesn't immediately need to triglycerides and transports them to fat cells for storage. Later, hormones regulate the release of triglycerides to meet your energy needs between meals. Just as you need some cholesterol for good health, you need a certain level of triglycerides. But high levels can be unhealthy. Most triglycerides are transported through your bloodstream as very-low-density lipoproteins.

How often should I have it done?

People who don't have diabetes should have a lipids test every 3 to 5 years — more often if their blood fat levels are above normal or they have a family history of elevated blood fats. People with diabetes should have the test at least once a year. That's because diabetes can accelerate the development of clogged and hardened arteries (atherosclerosis), which increases your risk of a heart attack, stroke and poor circulation in your feet and legs.

Is your blood fat where it should be at?

To help you evaluate your blood fat levels, here's a chart that shows what the National Heart, Lung and Blood Institute, a division of the National Institutes of Health, recommends for all Americans. These numbers are only guidelines. Each number takes on greater meaning when you look at it in relation to other health risk factors.

For people with diabetes, recommended HDL cholesterol and triglycerides levels are the same as those for all Americans. But the recommended LDL cholesterol level is lower. Because diabetes places you at greater risk of heart disease, the American Diabetes Association advocates an LDL cholesterol level of 100 milligrams per deciliter (mg/dL) of blood or lower.

	Recommended	Low risk	Borderline risk	High risk
LDL cholesterol	Less than 130 mg/dL **(For people with diabetes: 100 mg/dL or less)**	Less than 100 mg/dL	100-129 mg/dL	130 mg/dL or greater
HDL cholesterol	At least 35 mg/dL for men and 45 mg/dL for women	More than 45 mg/dL for men and 55 mg/dL for women	35-45 mg/dL for men and 45-55 mg/dL for women	Less than 35 mg/dL for men and 45 mg/dL for women
Triglycerides	Less than 200 mg/dL	Less than 200 mg/dL	200-399 mg/dL	400 mg/dL or more

How does it help?

A rising level of blood fats can alert your doctor to increased risk of blood vessel damage. Knowing your blood fat levels also helps your doctor determine if you could benefit from medication to lower your cholesterol or triglyceride levels. Diet and exercise are the first defenses against unhealthy blood fat levels, just as they are in managing diabetes. A cholesterol- or triglyceride-lowering medication may be prescribed if these steps aren't effective or if your LDL or triglyceride levels are extremely high.

Serum creatinine test

Diabetes can damage your kidneys' delicate filtering system that removes poisons from your body. A serum creatinine (kree-AT-i-nin) test can warn you of kidney problems. It measures the level of creatinine in your blood. Creatinine is a chemical waste product that's produced when you use your muscles. If your kidneys aren't functioning properly, they aren't able to remove this chemical from your blood.

Your blood normally contains a small amount of creatinine. If the results of your serum creatinine test are beyond the normal range, you may be experiencing kidney damage.

How often should I have it done?

You should have a serum creatinine test once a year. If you have known kidney damage, your doctor may recommend that you have this test more often.

How does it help?

Knowing the health of your kidneys is important because kidney function influences many decisions regarding your medical care, including which medications are safe for you to take and how aggressive to be in controlling your blood pressure.

Urine microalbumin test

A urine microalbumin test also is used to assess the health of your kidneys. But unlike the tests discussed previously, it's a urine test, not a blood test.

When your kidneys are functioning normally, they filter out only wastes in your blood, which you excrete in your urine. Protein and other helpful substances remain in the bloodstream. When your kidneys become damaged, the opposite occurs: Waste products remain in your blood and protein leaks into your urine.

When your kidneys first begin to leak, generally only small amounts of protein (albumin) escape. In the early stage of kidney disease, you may lose between 30 and 300 milligrams (mg) of albumin a day, a condition called microalbuminuria. A later and more advanced stage of the disease called macroalbuminuria (clinical proteinuria) generally occurs after you've had diabetes for 10 to 20 years. With macroalbuminuria, you're leaking more than 300 mg of albumin daily.

Various methods are used to screen for albumin leakage. The most reliable method is to save all of your urine over a 24-hour period in a clean jug that you get from your doctor. You then take the jug containing the urine to your doctor's office, where it's sent to a laboratory and analyzed. Recently developed screening methods require less urine. Laboratories can now detect excessive albumin excretion in the same amount of urine provided during routine urine testing (urinalysis).

How often should I have it done?

You should have a urine microalbumin test every year if:

- You've had type 1 diabetes for more than 5 years and you're past puberty.

- You have type 2 diabetes.

There's no 5-year wait with type 2 diabetes because the disease usually goes undiagnosed for many years. Unfortunately, many doctors don't routinely perform this test. One study reported that almost half of the more than 1,000 doctors surveyed didn't perform a microalbumin test on any of their patients with diabetes. If you haven't received the test, ask for it.

How does it help?

A urine microalbumin test can alert you and your doctor to kidney damage — hopefully while it's still in its early stages.

By keeping your blood sugar level within a normal or near-normal range, you can help prevent the progression of diabetes-related kidney disease. Controlling high blood pressure also is important in preventing further kidney damage. Blood pressure medications called angiotensin-converting enzyme (ACE) inhibitors often are prescribed to individuals with kidney damage because they help protect kidney function. Other classes of blood pressure medications also can be beneficial, and you may need more than one type. Eating a low-protein diet may improve protein leakage by reducing the workload on your kidneys. The typical American diet is high in protein — an average of 120 to 150 grams (g) a day. A low-protein diet contains less than 80 g of protein daily.

Questions and answers

Will exercising heavily or changing my diet a few days before a glycated hemoglobin test skew the results?
You can't alter the findings by altering your lifestyle a few days before the test. You can get an inaccurate reading, however, if you've had a recent blood transfusion or have experienced certain types of anemia.

Is one abnormal glycated hemoglobin test reason enough to change my treatment plan, or is it better to see if future tests also produce above-normal results?
One abnormal test definitely is reason to reassess your treatment plan. But this doesn't mean that your program needs to be changed completely. Perhaps just some modifications are in order. You may need to monitor your blood sugar more often, watch your diet more closely, get more physical activity or make dosage adjustments to your medications.

How much weight do I have to lose to improve my cholesterol?
Losing as little as 5 to 10 pounds can improve your cholesterol and triglyceride levels. Greater weight loss may bring even greater reductions.

What should I do if I feel that I'm not getting adequate follow-up care from my doctor?
Discuss your concerns regarding your treatment with your doctor. In areas where you're having problems or difficulties, ask him or her for suggestions on how to remedy them. If your doctor isn't

able to provide you with the information you need, ask to see another health professional who likely can: a diabetes specialist (endocrinologist), a diabetes physician extender, a diabetes educator or a registered dietitian. You should feel comfortable with the care you're receiving and have an open and positive rapport with your doctor and health care team.

Chapter 11

Self-care: Reducing your risk of complications

T reating your diabetes isn't a job that you can delegate solely to your doctor. It takes teamwork. Your health care team can supply you with a lot of helpful advice, information and care, but it's up to you to follow through. You're in the driver's seat.

It's also important that you approach your disease proactively instead of reactively. You want to prevent complications rather than simply respond to them when they occur. The following steps can help reduce detours in your treatment, improving your chances for a smooth ride ahead.

Have a yearly physical

Beyond your regular checkups to monitor your diabetes treatment, once a year have a thorough physical examination. As is typical of an annual physical, this is an examination from head to toe. The difference is that your doctor knows that you have diabetes and will be looking for emerging problems caused by the disease. An annual physical is an opportunity to screen for conditions, such as kidney or heart disease, which may not be part of your regular diabetes checkups. In addition, you may be so focused on your diabetes that you don't notice signs and symptoms associated with another condition. During an annual physical these features may come to light.

If you have a family or primary care doctor, he or she would be a good person to perform a physical examination. Your diabetes specialist also may serve as your primary care physician, particularly if you have type 1 diabetes.

Get a yearly eye exam

If you wait for vision problems to develop before you see an eye specialist, you've waited too long. Typically, by the time symptoms emerge, some permanent damage has already occurred. It's important to see an eye specialist (ophthalmologist or optometrist) annually to catch diabetes-related vision problems early, when they can still be treated. Make sure this person knows you have diabetes and performs a thorough examination, including dilation of your pupils. If your diabetes is poorly controlled, you have high blood pressure or kidney disease, or are pregnant, you may need to see an eye specialist more than once a year.

A thorough eye examination generally includes the following tests and procedures:

Visual acuity test. A visual acuity test determines your level of vision and need for corrective lenses, and it establishes a baseline measurement for future examinations.

External eye exam. An external eye exam measures your eye movements, along with the size of your pupils and their ability to respond to light.

Retinal exam. When doing a retinal exam, your eye specialist places medicated eyedrops into your eyes to dilate your pupils and check for damage to your retinas and the tiny blood vessels that nourish them. This is an especially important test because retinal damage is the most common eye complication of diabetes.

Glaucoma test. A glaucoma test (tonometry) measures the pressure in your eyes, which helps detect glaucoma, a disease that can gradually narrow your field of vision and produce tunnel vision and blindness. Diabetes increases your risk of developing glaucoma.

Slit-lamp exam. During a slit-lamp exam, your eye specialist evaluates the structures of your eyes, such as the cornea and iris.

He or she also looks for cataracts, which cloud your lenses and can make you feel as if you're looking through wax paper or a smudgy window. Diabetes can spur cataracts to develop sooner than they otherwise would.

Eye photography. If you have eye damage or suspected damage, photos may be taken with specially designed cameras to document the status of your vision and establish a baseline for future examinations.

See your dentist regularly

High blood sugar can impair your immune system from fighting off bacteria and viruses that cause infection. One common site of infection is your gums. That's because your mouth harbors many bacteria. If these germs settle in your gums and cause an infection, you may end up with gum disease that can cause your teeth to loosen and fall out.

To help prevent damage to your gums and teeth:

- See your dentist twice a year, and make sure he or she knows that you have diabetes.
- Brush your teeth twice a day.
- Floss every day.
- Look for early signs of gum disease, such as bleeding gums, redness and swelling. If you notice them, see your dentist.

Keep up-to-date on your vaccinations

Because high blood sugar can weaken your immune system, you may be more prone to getting influenza and pneumonia — and experience more serious effects — than people who don't have diabetes. If you have heart or kidney disease, you're at even higher risk of influenza or pneumonia.

Annual flu shot

The best way to avoid influenza or to reduce its symptoms is to have an annual flu shot (influenza vaccination). Get the shot before each flu season, which starts in about October in the Northern Hemisphere and April in the Southern Hemisphere. In the tropics you can catch influenza year-round.

In the United States, flu shots are modified annually to protect you against those influenza strains most likely to circulate during the coming winter. The vaccine contains only noninfectious viruses and can't cause the flu. The most common side effect is a little soreness at the spot where the injection is given. Although limited, some risks are associated with the vaccinations. Therefore it's a good idea to talk to your doctor before receiving one.

Pneumonia vaccine

Most doctors recommend people with diabetes receive a pneumonia vaccination. Depending on your age, you may need one or two injections. The Centers for Disease Control and Prevention recommends just one vaccination for people age 65 or older. If you're younger than 65 when you receive the vaccine, get a second vaccination (a booster shot) 5 years later.

The pneumonia vaccine contains antigens — substances that activate your immune system — that protect you against 85 percent to 90 percent of all forms of pneumonia found in the United States. Some people who receive the vaccine develop side effects similar to the flu. The effects generally last no more than 2 days.

Others

Make sure you're up-to-date on other important immunizations, such as a tetanus shot and its 10-year boosters. You may want to ask your doctor about getting vaccinated for protection against hepatitis B if you haven't received the vaccine already.

Care for your feet

Diabetes can cause two potentially dangerous threats to your feet: It can damage the nerves in your feet, and it can reduce blood flow to your feet. When the network of nerves in your feet is damaged, the sensation of pain in your feet is reduced. Because of this, you can develop a blister or cut your foot without realizing it. Diabetes also can narrow your arteries, reducing blood flow to your feet. With less blood to nourish tissues in your feet, it's harder for sores to heal. An unnoticed cut or sore hidden beneath your socks and shoes can quickly develop into a larger problem.

Check your feet every day

Use your eyes and hands to examine your feet. If you can't see some parts of your feet, use a mirror or ask your spouse, a family member or a friend to examine those locations. Look for the following:

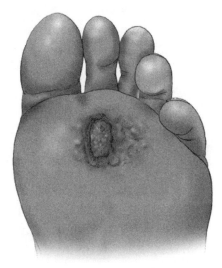

- Blisters, cuts and bruises

- Cracking, peeling and wrinkling

- Redness, red streaks and swelling

- Feet that are pinker, paler, darker or redder than usual, possibly due to pressure from tight shoes

Diabetes can impair blood circulation and nerve supply to your feet. Without proper attention and care, a small injury can develop into an open sore (ulcer) that can be difficult to treat.

Keep your feet clean and dry

Wash your feet each day with lukewarm water. To avoid burning your feet, test the water temperature with a thermometer. It should be no warmer than 90 F (32 C). Or test the water by touching a dampened washcloth to a sensitive area of your body, such as your face, neck or wrist.

Wash your feet with a gentle, massagelike motion, using a soft washcloth or sponge and a mild soap. Dry your skin by blotting or patting. Don't rub because you may rub too hard and accidentally damage your skin. Dry carefully between your toes to help prevent fungal infection.

Moisturize your skin

When diabetes damages your nerves, you may sweat less than normal, leaving your skin dry, especially on your feet. Dry skin can itch and crack, increasing your risk of an infection. To prevent dry skin use a moisturizer regularly.

Wear clean, dry socks

Wear socks made of fibers that pull (wick) sweat away from your skin. Avoid those with tight elastic bands that reduce circulation or that are thick or bulky. Bulky socks often fit poorly, and a poor fit can irritate your skin. It's also a good idea to avoid mended socks with thick seams that can rub and irritate your skin. Indentations from the seams in socks aren't a problem for most people, but among people with diabetes they can cause pressure sores.

Trim your toenails carefully

Bathe your feet in warm water and clean your toes carefully using a soft toothbrush and mild soap. Then cut the nails straight across so that they are even with the end of your toe. File rough edges so you don't have any sharp areas that could cut the neighboring toe. Be especially careful not to injure the surrounding skin. If you notice redness around the nails, report this to your regular doctor or your podiatrist.

Consulting a podiatrist

Because foot care is especially important to people with diabetes, your primary care doctor or diabetes specialist may recommend that you see a podiatrist. A podiatrist is a doctor who specializes in foot care. A podiatrist can teach you how to trim your toenails properly. If you have vision problems or significant loss of sensation in your feet, he or she can trim them for you.

A podiatrist also can teach you how to buy properly fitted shoes and prevent problems such as corns and calluses. If problems do occur, a podiatrist can help treat them to prevent more serious conditions from developing. Even small sores can quickly turn into serious problems without proper treatment.

Use foot products cautiously
Don't use a file or scissors on calluses, corns or bunions. You can injure your feet that way. Also, don't put chemicals on your feet, such as wart removers. See your regular doctor or podiatrist for problem calluses, corns, bunions or warts.

Wear shoes to protect your feet from injury
To help prevent injury to your feet and toes:

Always wear shoes. Around the house wear sturdy slippers.

Check your shoes. Look inside your shoes for tears or rough edges that might injure your feet. Shake out your shoes before you put them on to make sure nothing is inside, such as a pebble.

Select a comfortable and safe style of shoe. Good shoe design features include:

- Soft leather tops. Leather adapts to the shape of your foot and lets air circulate. Good air circulation reduces sweating, a major cause of skin irritation.

- Closed-toe design. Shoes with closed toes provide the best protection.

- Low-heeled shoes. These shoes are safer, more comfortable and less damaging to your feet.

- Flexible soles made from crepe or foam rubber. These soles are most comfortable for daily wear. They also act as good shock absorbers. Soles should provide solid footing and not be slippery.

Have at least two pairs of shoes so that you can switch shoes each day. This gives your shoes time to completely dry out and regain their shape. Don't wear wet shoes because moisture can shrink the material and make your shoes rub against your feet.

See your doctor if a problem develops
Even people who take great care of their feet sometimes develop foot sores. Obviously, you don't want to run to the doctor's office for every little nick or bruise on your feet. Most of these should

begin to heal within a couple of days to weeks. But if a wound isn't healing, appears to be getting bigger or looks as if it may be infected, see your regular doctor or podiatrist.

Does the shoe fit?

When you purchase new shoes:

- Make sure the tip of each shoe extends at least a quarter inch beyond your longest toe. The shoe tip also should be wide and long enough that your toes aren't cramped. Walk around the store with both of the new shoes on.

- If possible, try on shoes in the afternoon or evening. Your feet are more likely to swell this time of day, and you want shoes that are big enough to allow for normal swelling.

- If one foot is bigger than the other, buy shoes to fit your larger foot.

- If you have reduced sensation in your feet, don't rely on how the shoes feel on your feet. Take them home and wear them for 30 minutes, then remove them and examine your feet. Red areas indicate pressure and a poor fit. If you see any red areas, return the shoes. If no problems occur, gradually increase the time you wear them by $1/2$ to 1 hour each day.

Don't smoke

If you have diabetes and you smoke, you're three times more likely than nonsmokers with diabetes to die of heart disease or stroke, and you're more likely to develop circulation problems in your feet.

- Smoking narrows and hardens your arteries, reducing blood flow to your legs, making it more difficult for wounds to heal and increasing your risk of heart attack and stroke.

- Smoking increases your risk of nerve damage and kidney disease.

- Smoking appears to impair your immune system, producing more colds and respiratory infections.

If you're among the approximately 1 in 4 Americans with diabetes who smoke, talk to your doctor about methods to quit smoking. And don't be discouraged if your first attempts aren't successful. Stopping smoking can take several attempts.

Take a daily aspirin

The American Diabetes Association (ADA) recommends that most people with diabetes take an aspirin every day because studies show that daily aspirin use can reduce your risk of heart attack by up to 60 percent. The recommended dose is anywhere from 81 milligrams (mg) a day, the amount found in a baby aspirin, to 325 mg a day, the amount in an adult tablet.

When you have diabetes, you produce more "sticky" platelets that attach themselves to the inside walls of your arteries, clogging your arteries and causing blood clots to form. Clogged arteries and blood clots can lead to a heart attack or a stroke. Aspirin is an anti-clotting, antiplatelet drug that decreases the stickiness of your platelets, reducing your risk of narrowed arteries or blood clots.

It's best to take aspirin with food and to take coated aspirin tablets that dissolve in your small intestine instead of your stomach. A serious side effect of regular aspirin usage is that it can cause stomach irritation, bleeding or an ulcer. Once you start taking aspirin, you may notice that you bruise more easily and the bruises last longer. That's because aspirin reduces the ability of your blood platelets to seal up and heal wounds.

Aspirin therapy, however, isn't for everyone. Aspirin isn't recommended for children because it can produce a dangerous condition called Reye's syndrome. You also shouldn't take aspirin if:

- You've had an allergic reaction to aspirin in the past.
- You have a stomach ulcer.
- You have liver disease.
- You're taking some other drug that reduces clotting, such as warfarin (Coumadin).

If you can't take aspirin and your doctor considers you at high risk of a heart attack or stroke, he or she may recommend a prescription blood-thinning medication.

Monitor your blood pressure

People with diabetes are twice as likely to develop high blood pressure as individuals who don't have diabetes. If you're black, your chances of having both diabetes and high blood pressure are double that of a white person. If you're Hispanic, that chance triples.

Whatever your race, having both diabetes and high blood pressure is serious. Like diabetes, high blood pressure can damage your blood vessels. When these two conditions team up, they can undermine your health and produce a heart attack, a stroke or any number of other life-threatening conditions. Between 35 percent and 75 percent of all complications associated with diabetes can be attributed to having high blood pressure.

Blood pressure is a measure of the force of circulating blood against the walls of your arteries. The higher your blood pressure, the harder your heart has to work to pump blood to all parts of your body. Blood pressure is measured as two numbers, such as 120/70 millimeters of mercury (mm Hg). The first number (upper number) is the systolic pressure, your peak pressure at the moment your heart contracts and pumps blood. The second number (lower number) is the diastolic pressure, the level of pressure when your heart relaxes to allow blood to flow into your heart. The ADA recommends that adults with diabetes keep their blood pressure below 130/85 mm Hg. If you have kidney disease, your doctor may recommend a lower blood pressure.

The same healthy habits that can improve your blood sugar — a balanced diet and regular exercise — can help reduce your blood pressure. Limiting consumption of sodium also is important. If you can't control your blood pressure with diet and exercise alone, your doctor may prescribe blood pressure-lowering medication. The drugs most commonly used for people with diabetes are angiotensin-converting enzyme (ACE) inhibitors or angiotensin II receptor blockers. These medications have a low rate of side effects, and they help protect your kidneys and heart, which are at high risk of damage from both diseases. Other high blood pressure medications prescribed to people with diabetes include diuretics, beta blockers, calcium antagonists and alpha blockers.

You should have your blood pressure checked at every doctor visit. If you have high blood pressure — especially if it's not well controlled — you may also want to monitor your blood pressure regularly at home.

Manage stress

When you're under a lot of stress, it can become more difficult to take good care of yourself and your diabetes. You might not eat right. You may not exercise. And you may not take your medication as prescribed. Excessive or prolonged stress also can increase production of hormones that block the effect of insulin, causing your blood sugar to rise.

If stress is a problem for you, stop and think about what causes you stress. Then ask yourself if you can do anything to change the situation. If a hectic day of running from one event to another stresses you out, reduce your daily commitments. If certain friends, neighbors or family members cause you stress, limit the time you spend with them. If your job is stressful, look for ways to lighten the load, such as handing over some of your responsibilities to others. You also can ask your health care team for advice. Some basic stress-fighting techniques include:

Eating a balanced diet. Eating a variety of nutrients keeps all of your body's systems working and gives you strength to cope with stressful situations.

Exercising regularly. Exercise burns off nervous energy and gives you strength.

Getting adequate sleep. A good night's sleep refreshes you so that you're ready to tackle the day's problems.

Relief through relaxation

You can't avoid all of the stress that comes your way, but you can minimize the effects of stress by learning healthy ways to relax when you're feeling stressed. There are many methods of relaxation. Some people relax while listening to or performing music. Others surround themselves with soothing aromas (aromatherapy). Still others benefit from practices such as yoga or meditation.

To help you get started, here are two simple relaxation techniques you can use when you begin to feel stressed:

Deep breathing. Most adults breathe from their chest. Each time you breathe in (inhale) your chest expands. Each time you breathe out (exhale) it contracts. To relax, breathe deeply from your diaphragm, the muscle that separates the chest from the abdomen. You can use deep breathing as your only means of relaxation or as a warm-up and cool-down method for other techniques.

Taking a breather

Here's an exercise to help you practice deep, relaxed breathing. Rehearse it throughout the day until you can automatically apply it when you feel stressed:

- Sit comfortably with your feet flat on the floor.
- Loosen tight clothing around your abdomen and waist.
- Place your hands on your lap or at your side.
- Close your eyes if doing so helps you to relax.
- Breathe in slowly through your nose while counting to four. Allow your abdomen to expand as you breathe in.
- Pause for a second and then exhale at a normal rate through your mouth.
- Repeat until you feel more relaxed.

Progressive muscle relaxation. This technique involves relaxing a series of muscles one at a time. First, raise the tension level in a group of muscles, such as a leg or an arm, by tightening the muscles and then relaxing them. Concentrate on slowly letting the tension go in each muscle. Then move on to the next muscle group.

Questions and answers

I like to travel. Can I do so safely with diabetes?

There's no reason you can't travel. The key is to make sure that you're well-prepared. Carry medical identification with you and bring enough diabetes supplies and medications to last the entire trip — plus a little extra in case of scheduling changes. Don't put these items in checked bags. Keep them in your carry-on bag. When making your reservations, you can request a special diabetic meal. Also take along food such as dried fruits or crackers to treat low blood sugar or in case you don't eat on schedule. Pack two pairs of good walking shoes, should you have problems with one pair. As much as possible, try to follow your daily walking and eating regimen.

Will another pain reliever such as Tylenol or Advil reduce my risk of a heart attack?

No. Like aspirin, acetaminophen and ibuprofen help reduce pain. But they don't have aspirin's anticlotting capabilities.

I was told that because I have diabetes, I should avoid sitting with my legs crossed. Why?

Crossing your legs increases pressure on the nerves in your legs and may increase nerve damage.

Should I join a support group for people with diabetes?

Many people find support groups helpful. You might consider joining a support group if you don't have a knowledgeable, understanding and supportive group of family and friends to help you. You also might join a support group if you feel that you could benefit from encouragement and coping strategies members can offer. However, support groups aren't for everyone. Some people find it difficult or intimidating to interact within groups. If you would like to learn more about support groups, talk with your doctor, diabetes educator or dietitian. Another good source of support is the American Diabetes Association (see page 185).

Thank you for purchasing Mayo Clinic on Managing Diabetes!

We hope you enjoy your book. Please take a few minutes to complete this questionnaire. Your input will help us develop other books and products. We also can inform you of products that might be of interest to you.

As our way of saying thanks, we will send you a free issue of one of our highly acclaimed newsletters: *Mayo Clinic Health Letter* or *Mayo Clinic Women's HealthSource.* Please select **one** of the newsletters below:

☐ *Mayo Clinic Health Letter* is a monthly 8-page newsletter that covers general health issues and provides information you can use to live a healthier life.

☐ *Mayo Clinic Women's HealthSource* is a monthly 8-page newsletter that is devoted entirely to the special health interests of women.

Thank you for your time.

Tell us where to send your FREE newsletter issue:

© Mayo Foundation for Medical Education and Research

1. Which of these health topics are you interested in? *(Please select up to 5 topics.)*
- ☐ Allergies or asthma
- ☐ Alzheimer's / memory disorders
- ☐ Arthritis
- ☐ Breast cancer
- ☐ Chronic pain
- ☐ Colon cancer
- ☐ Depression
- ☐ Diabetes
- ☐ Digestive diseases
- ☐ Eye or vision problems
- ☐ Hearing loss
- ☐ Heart disease
- ☐ High blood pressure
- ☐ Impotence or erectile dysfunction
- ☐ Insomnia or other sleep disorders
- ☐ Lung cancer
- ☐ Menopause
- ☐ Migraines or other headaches
- ☐ Pregnancy
- ☐ Prostate problems
- ☐ Stroke

2. Which of the following lifestyle topics are you interested in?
- ☐ Alternative medicine
- ☐ Exercise and fitness
- ☐ Healthy cooking
- ☐ Healthy aging
- ☐ Healthy weight
- ☐ Nutrition
- ☐ Skin care
- ☐ Stress management
- ☐ Vitamins, minerals or herbs

3. Where did you purchase this book?
- ☐ Book club
- ☐ Bookstore
- ☐ Discount store (e.g., *Kmart, Target*)
- ☐ Drugstore
- ☐ Grocery store
- ☐ Internet
- ☐ Mail order
- ☐ Phone order
- ☐ Retail store
- ☐ Warehouse store (*Sam's Club, etc.*)

4. What sources do you use to get health information?
- ☐ Books
- ☐ Internet
- ☐ Magazines
- ☐ Newsletters
- ☐ Television
- ☐ Other

5. Do you have access to the Internet?
☐ Yes ☐ No

Name _____

Address _____ Apt _____

City _____ State _____ Zip _____

E-mail Address _____

MC2011-44

BUSINESS REPLY MAIL
FIRST-CLASS MAIL   PERMIT NO. 251   ROCHESTER MN

POSTAGE WILL BE PAID BY ADDRESSEE

MAYO CLINIC HEALTH INFORMATION
CENTERPLACE 5
200 1ST ST SW
ROCHESTER MN   55902-9826

NO POSTAGE
NECESSARY
IF MAILED
IN THE
UNITED STATES

Chapter 12

Sexual health: Issues for women and men

S exuality is an important part of your overall well-being and another aspect of your health influenced by diabetes. Understanding how diabetes affects sexuality, and what you can do about it, can minimize the disease's effects and help you lead a more enjoyable life.

If you're a woman, knowing that fluctuations in your hormone levels may affect your blood sugar (glucose) can help you better manage your diabetes during menstruation and menopause. If you're considering pregnancy, key steps before and during your pregnancy can greatly improve your chances for delivering a healthy baby, without complications.

If you're a man, the better you control your blood sugar, the less your risk of impotence due to nerve and blood vessel damage. If you're already experiencing impotence, treatments are available.

Some people find it difficult to discuss sexual matters. But it's important to ask your doctor questions if you have concerns or are experiencing problems.

Menstruation and blood sugar

Estrogen and progesterone are hormones produced by your ovaries that regulate your reproductive cycle. As their levels fluctuate during the month, so can your blood sugar level.

The first 2 weeks of your menstrual cycle begin at the onset of vaginal bleeding. During this time estrogen and progesterone levels are low, and they slowly rise as your ovaries ripen an egg for ovulation and fertilization. Near the third week of your menstrual cycle, estrogen production increases as the egg is released into your fallopian tubes, which lead to your uterus. Production of progesterone also increases, preparing the lining of your uterus for pregnancy. If the egg isn't fertilized, your ovaries stop producing estrogen and progesterone, which causes menstruation, the shedding of the blood and tissue that line your uterus.

Reproductive hormones and blood sugar

Estrogen typically makes your cells more responsive to insulin. So when the amount of estrogen in your body increases, your blood sugar level may drop. Progesterone, on the other hand, makes your cells more resistant to insulin. As progesterone production increases, your blood sugar levels may rise.

Production of these two hormones varies throughout the menstrual cycle and doesn't always occur simultaneously or to the same degree. The majority of women who monitor their blood sugar levels don't notice a significant change in them. Women who do experience fluctuations may be influenced by other factors that can accompany menstruation, such as variations in their diet or level of physical activity.

It's generally during the third week of your menstrual cycle, at the time of ovulation, that estrogen and progesterone levels are highest and you're most likely to experience changes in your blood sugar. These changes tend to be more noticeable or dramatic in women with premenstrual syndrome (PMS). Premenstrual syndrome is a condition that occurs in some women about a week before menstruation. Symptoms include mood swings, tender breasts, bloating, lethargy, food cravings and lack of concentration. Giving in to cravings for carbohydrates and fats also can make blood sugar control more difficult.

High blood sugar also can lead to other sexual problems such as:

- A dry vagina
- Yeast infections of the vagina
- Irregular menstrual periods
- Decreased lubrication during sexual intercourse
- Loss of skin sensation around the vaginal area

How to respond

To respond to blood sugar variations caused by hormonal fluctuations, record your blood sugar levels on a daily basis. Note any symptoms you experience before menstruation, such as bloating, irritability, fatigue, cramps, weight gain or food cravings. Also record the day your period begins and the day it ends. Look for patterns in your blood sugar levels, especially the week before your period.

If your blood sugar levels are higher than normal before your period, you may need to make an adjustment in your treatment program. You might ask your doctor about gradually increasing your dose of insulin to coincide with the days of your blood sugar elevations. Any change in your medication needs to be done under the guidance of your doctor. You'll want to return to your usual dose of insulin as soon as your period begins. Other strategies to help offset a temporary increase in blood sugar include increasing the amount you exercise and modifying your diet.

If your blood sugar levels are lower than normal before your period, you might ask your doctor about adjusting your insulin dose — in this case, lowering it — a few days before your period begins. Alternatives to altering your medication include reducing, but not eliminating, the amount you exercise and eating more carbohydrates. But don't load up on junk food.

Making it through menopause

Near age 40 many women begin to experience symptoms of perimenopause, changes that occur around (peri) the end of menstruation (menopause). During perimenopause estrogen and progesterone levels often fluctuate as your body prepares for menopause, which generally occurs between the ages of 45 and 55. Perimenopausal symptoms, such as hot flashes, missed periods, mood changes and sleep difficulties, are associated with lower levels of estrogen, but the exact cause of the symptoms is unknown.

Effects on blood sugar during this time are varied and inconsistent. Because your body is maturing fewer eggs, your ovaries produce less estrogen. As estrogen levels decline, your blood sugar levels may rise due to an increased resistance to insulin. Production of progesterone also declines during this period. Lower amounts of progesterone have the opposite effect. They can cause your blood sugar levels to drop because of increased sensitivity to insulin.

According to the American Diabetes Association, when menopause is complete, most women with diabetes require approximately 20 percent less medication — oral medications or insulin — to control their diabetes because their cells are more sensitive to insulin. However, this may be offset by changes that can occur after menopause, such as weight gain. Additional weight increases your cells' resistance to insulin and may increase your need for medication.

How to respond

Your best response to blood sugar changes that can accompany perimenopause and menopause is to monitor your blood sugar regularly and make adjustments to correspond with the changes.

Many women find perimenopausal and menopausal discomforts to be minimal and can control their symptoms with self-help strategies, such as additional exercise and changes in their diet. For women with more severe symptoms, some doctors recommend oral contraceptives or hormone replacement therapy to help control hormonal fluctuations.

Hormone replacement therapy

Hormone replacement therapy (HRT) helps ease troublesome symptoms of menopause for many women. It also can reduce the risk of osteoporosis and heart disease, and there's some evidence that HRT may protect against Alzheimer's disease.

The most common form of HRT provides supplemental estrogen and progesterone, which are nearly nonexistent in a woman's body following menopause. The medication is typically prescribed after you experience your first hot flash or other discomforts due to menopausal symptoms.

Different HRT regimens are available. They vary according to the type of estrogen and progesterone preparations used, doses of the hormones and the form of administration. HRT is most commonly taken in pill form but also is available as a patch or a cream. In addition, the regimen may be cyclic or continuous. A cyclic method provides estrogen daily and a progestational preparation (progestin) 10 to 14 days of the month. This usually leads to monthly vaginal bleeding. A continuous method provides low doses of estrogen and progestin daily and may cause more irregular bleeding.

Is it OK to take HRT?

Whether to take HRT is an individual decision, based on each woman's health history and health risks. Visit with your doctor about HRT to see if it's a good choice for you. You'll want to consider these factors:

Blood sugar. The effect of HRT on your blood sugar depends on the treatment method you choose and whether you experienced variations in your blood sugar during your menstrual cycle. If you experienced fluctuations before menopause, you may be more likely to experience fluctuations with use of HRT.

Heart disease. Diabetes increases a woman's risk of a heart attack or stroke, especially following menopause, when estrogen production decreases. A postmenopausal woman who has diabetes is three times more likely to experience a heart attack or stroke than a postmenopausal woman who doesn't have diabetes.

Studies suggest that HRT can lower your risk of developing heart disease. This observation is likely a result of multiple changes associated with estrogen therapy, including the lowering of "bad" low-density lipoprotein (LDL) cholesterol and the raising of "good" high-density lipoprotein (HDL) cholesterol. Ongoing studies on the effects of HRT should provide more definitive answers regarding HRT use and heart disease risk. If you already have heart disease, studies indicate that beginning HRT isn't beneficial. It doesn't protect you against future cardiac events.

Osteoporosis. Hormone replacement therapy slows the loss of calcium from your bones after menopause. Combined with regular exercise and adequate calcium, it protects against loss of bone mass and reduces your risk of fractures.

Cancer. Use of HRT has been linked to an increased risk of breast cancer, especially among women who use HRT for more than 5 years. Most of this information is based on observational studies, and it hasn't been proved in clinical trials. Results of an ongoing study called the Women's Health Initiative should provide more concrete data on HRT use and the risk of breast cancer. These results should be available in 4 to 5 years. It's also important to remember that even though HRT is linked to an increased risk of breast cancer, despite the increase, for many women their overall risk of developing breast cancer is still quite low, in the absence of other risk factors.

Uterine cancer is another risk associated with HRT use. This cancer is more common among women taking estrogen alone who haven't had a hysterectomy. Combining progesterone with estrogen offers some protection against uterine cancer.

Diabetes and pregnancy

There was a time when women with diabetes were told not to become pregnant. If they did, their babies often didn't survive. Even after insulin became available in the early 1920s, the number of successful pregnancies in women with diabetes remained much lower than in women without diabetes.

Today, the chances of a woman with diabetes having a normal pregnancy are almost the same as for a woman without diabetes. The reason? Intensive (tight) blood sugar control before conception and throughout pregnancy.

It's important to make the distinction between type 1 and 2 diabetes and gestational diabetes. Unlike type 1 and 2 diabetes, which develop before or after pregnancy, gestational diabetes occurs during pregnancy, generally in the second or third trimester. This form of diabetes is caused by increased production of the hormones estrogen and progesterone that occurs during pregnancy. Gestational diabetes also differs in that it disappears immediately following delivery. Having gestational diabetes does increase your risk of developing type 2 diabetes. More than half of women who experience gestational diabetes develop type 2 disease later in life.

Rarely, some women develop type 1 diabetes during pregnancy. In most cases, the condition is initially diagnosed as gestational diabetes. But unlike gestational diabetes, blood sugar levels don't improve following birth of the baby. They remain high and require insulin to control them.

Blood sugar and your baby's health

Blood sugar control is very important to the health of an unborn baby. During the first 8 weeks of development — when the baby's heart, lungs, kidneys and brain are being formed — if the mother's blood sugar is too high, the fetus is at increased risk of birth defects or miscarriage. A high blood acid level (diabetic ketoacidosis) also can cause miscarriage.

Later in pregnancy, uncontrolled blood sugar can lead to premature birth or stillbirth. Excess blood sugar also can cause the baby to grow larger than normal and make delivery more complicated. Opposite of the mother, the baby may be born with a low blood sugar level. Another possible complication is a yellowish skin color (jaundice) from buildup of old blood cells that aren't being cleared away fast enough by the baby's liver. Fortunately, both conditions are easily treatable.

Risks to the mother from uncontrolled blood sugar during pregnancy include high blood pressure and a worsening of pre-existing diabetes complications, especially eye disease (retinopathy).

Planning your pregnancy

To prevent diabetes-related complications to you and your fetus, it's crucial that you be in control of your blood sugar before you

Intensive insulin therapy reduces birth defects

Studies by the American Diabetes Association show that among women with type 1 diabetes who begin a program of intensive insulin therapy (tight blood sugar control) before conception, only 1 percent of babies experience birth defects, compared with 10 percent of babies born to mothers who begin intensive insulin therapy after conception. Intensive therapy involves frequent adjustments to your insulin doses to maintain normal blood sugar levels.

The changes your body goes through during pregnancy affect your blood sugar level and make controlling diabetes more difficult. As your pregnancy progresses, the placenta produces hormones that decrease insulin's ability to lower blood sugar. This means you may require two or three times the amount of insulin you normally take, and you may need to give yourself insulin injections more often. Always check with your doctor before making any changes to your insulin regimen.

become pregnant. A diabetes management plan, developed with the guidance of your doctor and health care team, can help you achieve good blood sugar control and prepare your body for a healthy pregnancy.

This plan generally includes the following:

Use of birth control. Practicing birth control before pregnancy allows you to choose the safest and most appropriate time to have a child. If you use oral contraception (birth control pills), Depo-Provera (injections) or Norplant (surgically inserted tubes) for birth control, you may need to adjust your insulin regimen.

When your glycated hemoglobin (hemoglobin A-1C) test reaches near-normal levels, your doctor may recommend discontinuing birth control. This test is an overall measurement of your blood sugar. See Chapter 10 for more information on the glycated hemoglobin test.

A complete physical examination. A physical examination helps to identify potential risks for pregnancy-related complications, such as high blood pressure, and eye, nerve or kidney disease. Because pregnancy may worsen diabetic problems, it's important to treat these conditions before becoming pregnant.

Regular blood sugar monitoring. Consistently monitoring your blood sugar level is one of the most important things you can do to reduce the risk of diabetes-related complications to you and your baby. Before and after you become pregnant, your doctor will encourage you to test your blood sugar several times each day and adjust your insulin dose accordingly. You'll want to check your blood sugar level before each meal, 1 to 2 hours after each meal and at bedtime. Your doctor may even recommend that you check your blood sugar during the middle of the night.

Meal planning. A healthy meal plan helps you maintain normal or near-normal blood sugar levels. You may need to work with a dietitian to modify your meal plan to address problems with pregnancy, including nausea and vomiting, constipation or food cravings.

Artificial sweeteners are a concern for mothers with diabetes. The effects of saccharin on the fetus are unknown, so it's best during your pregnancy to avoid products containing saccharin. Aspartame, made of aspartate and phenylalanine, doesn't seem to cause problems. Still it's best to consume in moderation products containing aspartame.

Regular exercise. Years ago, women with diabetes were advised not to exercise during pregnancy because of concerns that exercise might affect the health of the baby. Today, doctors recommend all people exercise daily to improve their health, including women with diabetes who are pregnant. It's important to test your blood sugar before and after you exercise to avoid low blood sugar.

Preventing potential problems

Tight blood sugar control can help prevent complications of pregnancy, but tight control also puts you at risk of low blood sugar (hypoglycemia). Your body gets used to your blood sugar being between a certain, narrow range. When your blood sugar drops below that range, your body, in a sense, overreacts. Warning signs of low blood sugar include shaking, sweating, clumsy movements, confusion, headache, hunger, paleness and mood and behavior changes. Possible causes of low blood sugar include too much exercise, too much insulin, not enough food and not eating on time.

High blood sugar (hyperglycemia), another potential problem of tight control, can occur if your body doesn't have enough insulin, you overeat or you exercise less than you planned. Stress or illness, such as a cold or influenza, also may cause high blood sugar. Symptoms may include frequent urination, increased thirst and fatigue.

Diabetic ketoacidosis is another condition to be aware of. It's caused by increased levels of ketones, a blood acid that results when your cells lack sugar and your body begins to break down fat for energy. Ketones, a byproduct of fat metabolism, can build up in your blood and become dangerous to your health — and the baby's. For more on these conditions, see Chapter 2.

During your pregnancy
Regular visits with members of your health care team can help you keep your diabetes management plan on track during your pregnancy.

First trimester. During the first 10 to 12 weeks of your pregnancy, you'll meet with your obstetrician regularly, perhaps every 1 to 2 weeks. This is the time that your baby's vital organs are developing, so you want your blood sugar to be as close to normal as possible. Frequent blood sugar monitoring can help you do this. Because

Your health care team

Achieving and maintaining blood sugar control during pregnancy is easier if you assemble a team of health care personnel familiar with diabetes. Such a team includes:

- Your diabetes specialist
- An obstetrician specializing in high-risk pregnancies and pregnancies of women with diabetes
- A pediatrician or neonatologist who can treat potential conditions of babies born to women with diabetes
- A registered dietitian and a diabetes educator experienced in teaching people how to achieve tight blood sugar control

your body's need for insulin may drop slightly during this time, it's important to be alert to signs of low blood sugar. If morning sickness makes you really miserable, talk with your doctor about use of anti-nausea medication.

Second trimester. The second trimester is when many pregnant women receive an ultrasound examination to check the health of the baby. Your doctor also will keep track of your weight gain. Over the course of your pregnancy, you should gain between 15 and 30 pounds, depending on your weight before you became pregnant. Overweight women should try to limit weight gain to 15 pounds. For women of normal weight, an increase of 20 to 30 pounds is often recommended.

If you take insulin, expect your insulin requirements to rise gradually to about week 20 and then accelerate dramatically. Hormones made by the placenta to help the baby grow block the effect of the mother's insulin. As a result your insulin needs increase significantly. At this stage of your pregnancy it's also important to see an eye specialist. Damage to small blood vessels in your eyes can progress during pregnancy because of additional hormones manufactured by the placenta.

Third trimester. As your pregnancy enters its final 3 months, your doctor will monitor you carefully for possible complications that can occur during the late stage of any pregnancy: high blood pressure, swollen ankles from fluid buildup and kidney problems. You may receive another ultrasound exam to assess the size and health of your baby. You also should have your eyes examined again to check for eye damage. At this stage, a potential problem to you or your baby may prompt early delivery of the baby.

Delivering your baby

Your health care team will help you determine the best time and safest method to deliver your baby. Delivering your baby at home with a nurse midwife generally isn't recommended because of the increased potential for problems due to your diabetes.

As long as your blood sugar remains normal and you or the baby aren't experiencing complications, you can expect a normal vaginal delivery. During labor it's important to monitor your blood sugar often to prevent a large reduction or increase in your blood sugar levels. Because your body is working so hard, you'll likely need less insulin. If there are complications, your baby may be delivered by Caesarean section (C-section) through an incision in your lower abdominal and uterine walls. Regardless of the delivery method, the result for most women who've maintained good blood sugar control is a healthy baby.

Following delivery of your baby, your insulin needs will decrease. However, it may take a few weeks to months before your body changes are complete and you return to your normal insulin regimen before becoming pregnant.

Dealing with impotence

More than half of men age 50 and older with diabetes experience some degree of impotence. But few of them talk about it with their doctors. This is too bad because if they did, chances are good their doctors could help them treat the condition.

Impotence refers to the inability to achieve an erection of the penis or to maintain an erection long enough for sexual intercourse. Another term commonly used to describe this condition is erectile dysfunction.

Impotence can result from physical or psychological factors. The most common causes in men with diabetes are physical problems due to poor blood sugar control or long-term effects of the disease. Excess blood sugar can damage the nerves and blood vessels responsible for erections. When the nerves are damaged, they're no longer able to communicate with small blood vessels in the penis, telling them to expand to accommodate the flow of blood necessary for an erection. When large blood vessels are narrowed or blocked, not enough blood reaches the penis to cause an erection.

Psychological factors that can produce impotence include anxiety, stress or depression. They can interfere with your body's normal production of hormones and the manner in which your brain responds to them, preventing erections from occurring. For some men, simply hearing about erectile problems associated with diabetes creates a fear of the condition that actually causes it to occur.

Certain medications also can cause impotence, including some drugs used to treat high blood pressure, anxiety and depression. If you're experiencing impotence, make sure your doctor is aware of all of the medications you take.

Several therapies are available to treat impotence. They may not be able to reverse, or cure, your condition, but they can make it possible for you to partake in sexual intercourse. Finding the treatment method that works best for you and that you're the most comfortable with may take time.

Medications

The first step in finding an effective treatment for impotence is often medication:

Sildenafil. For some men with impotence resulting from diabetes, the medication sildenafil (Viagra) can improve sexual function. But it isn't effective for everyone.

Unlike other treatments for impotence, sildenafil produces a natural erection instead of an artificial one. The drug helps you respond to sexual or psychological stimulation by relaxing the smooth muscle tissue in the penis, which in turn increases blood flow in the penis and makes it easier for you to achieve and maintain an erection. You take the blue, diamond-shaped tablet about an hour before sexual intercourse. The drug is effective for about 4 hours and shouldn't be used more than once a day.

Sildenafil isn't safe for all men. You shouldn't take the drug if you're also taking nitrates, such as nitroglycerin. Taken together, this mix of medicine can substantially lower your blood pressure and produce a fatal heart attack. Sildenafil can cause other side effects. It may produce facial flushing, which generally lasts no more than 5 to 10 minutes. You also may experience a temporary, mild headache or an upset stomach. Higher doses can produce short-term visual problems: a slight bluish tinge to objects, blurred vision and increased light sensitivity. These effects subside a few hours after taking the drug.

Alprostadil. Alprostadil is a synthetic version of the hormone prostaglandin E-1. Like sildenafil, this medication helps relax smooth muscle tissue in the penis, enhancing blood flow and causing an erection. Sometimes, alprostadil is combined with other vasodilator medications to improve its effects. Alprostadil is not a pill, rather it's delivered by suppository (self-intraurethral therapy) or by self-injection.

Self-intraurethral therapy. With self-intraurethral therapy, you place a rubber ring around the base of your penis and then use a disposable applicator to insert a tiny (about half the size of a grain of rice) suppository into the tip of your penis. The trade name of this alprostadil suppository is Muse. The suppository is absorbed by erectile tissue in your penis, increasing blood flow that causes an erection. The rubber ring helps trap the blood and maintain an erection.

Side effects may include some pain, dizziness and formation of hard, fibrous tissue. After a test dose in the doctor's office, you learn to perform the procedure yourself.

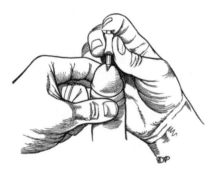

Self-intraurethral therapy involves injecting a tiny suppository into the tip of your penis to help relax smooth muscle tissue and increase blood flow to the penis.

Self-injection. With self-injection you use a fine needle to inject alprostadil into the base or side of your penis. Self-injected alprostadil (Caverject, Edex) increases blood flow into the sponge-like structures that run the length of your penis on each side, producing an erection. It generally takes 5 to 20 minutes for the drug to work, with the erection lasting about an hour. Because the needle is so thin — like those used to inject insulin — pain from the injection is usually minor.

Side effects may include bleeding from the injection and on rare occasions a prolonged, painful erection (priapism). To minimize the risk of a prolonged erection, it's important that you test the medication to determine the proper dose. If an erection continues for more than 4 hours, the blood trapped inside your penis becomes thick because of oxygen loss. This can damage tissue in your penis. Another rare side effect is the formation of a lump (fibrosis) at the injection site. This method can also cause bruising if you accidentally nick a small blood vessel with the needle.

Self-injection therapy involves injecting medication directly into a specific area of the penis to increase blood flow and cause an erection.

Vacuum devices

Many men turn to vacuum devices when medication is ineffective or its side effects are too bothersome. The devices use vacuum pressure to draw blood into your penis. You begin by placing a plastic tube over your penis. Using a hand pump, you draw air out of the plastic tube. As you do this, blood is pulled into the tissue of your penis, producing a strong erection. You then slip off an elastic ring mounted on the base of the plastic tube, pulling it onto the base of your penis. The ring traps the blood inside your penis, allowing you to keep your erection once the tube is removed. You should remove the ring within 30 minutes to restore normal blood flow to your penis. If you don't, you could damage penile tissue. A vacuum pump is effective in more than 90 percent of men who use it, and it doesn't require medication or surgery.

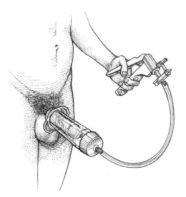

A vacuum device uses a hand pump to draw blood into the penis and create an erection. An elastic ring placed at the base of the penis keeps it erect.

Penile implants

If you've tried medication or a vacuum device and they haven't worked or have been uncomfortable, you might consider a surgical implant. There are three types:

Semirigid, bendable rod. A semirigid, bendable rod type of implant is the easiest to use and the least likely to malfunction. Two hard but flexible rods made of wires and covered with silicone or polyurethane are placed inside your penis. They give you a permanent erection. You bend your penis down toward your body to hide the erection and bend it up to have sexual intercourse. Though it looks unnatural and takes some getting used to, this implant requires less surgical time than other implants, it has no mechanical parts to break and it has a high success rate.

Inflatable. These implants work more naturally than the semirigid rods. Instead of having a permanent erection, you produce an erection only when you want one.

One version includes two hollow cylinders that are placed into your penis. These cylinders are connected to a tiny pump in your scrotum and to a reservoir in either your scrotum or your lower abdomen. When you squeeze the pump, fluid from the reservoir fills the cylinders and produces an erection. The device is easily concealed and very effective, but it's more likely than other implants to suffer mechanical failure.

Another version doesn't involve a pump. Instead, a device near the head of your penis controls the flow of fluid inside the cylinders. To get an erection, you squeeze the head of your penis.

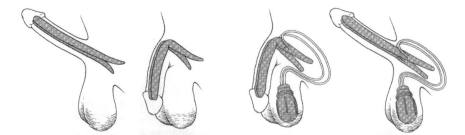

With a semirigid, bendable rod implant (left) the penis is always erect. To hide the erection, the penis is bent down. With inflatable implants (right), the implanted cylinders need to be inflated to achieve an erection.

This releases fluid into the cylinders. To shift the fluid back into place and produce a limp penis, you bend the implant and press a release valve.

Interlocking blocks. This type of implant is similar to the semi-rigid implant except that it contains a series of small blocks connected by a tiny steel cable. It's simple to use, easy to conceal and produces an erection only when you want one.

Counseling

If your impotence is related to psychological factors, the most effective form of treatment may be to meet with a therapist who is familiar with sexual issues. This may include a licensed psychiatrist, psychologist or counselor. Discussing your fears and concerns or, if you're depressed, identifying the source of your depression often is helpful in improving your sex life.

Questions and answers

Why does my blood sugar level drop following sexual intercourse?
Your body responds to sexual intercourse as it does exercise. Just as blood sugar drops during and following exercise due to increased need for energy (glucose) by your muscles and tissues, so it does with sexual intercourse. Testing your blood sugar before having sexual intercourse can save you an episode of low blood sugar afterward. To prevent a decrease in blood sugar, you might eat something beforehand or immediately afterward.

If I have diabetes, what are the chances that my child will develop it too?
A genetic counselor can help you predict the likelihood of having a child with type 1 or type 2 diabetes. According to the American Diabetes Association, for a child born to a mother age 25 or older with type 1 diabetes, the risk of having diabetes is about the same — 1 percent — as that of a child born to parents who don't have diabetes. The risk increases to about 4 percent if the mother is younger than age 25 when the child is born. If the father has type 1 diabetes, the risk increases to about 6 percent. If either parent developed type 1 diabetes before age 11, the risk doubles.

Type 2 diabetes, on the other hand, tends to run in families. Lifestyle habits related to food and exercise may be more likely than genetics to influence whether your child develops type 2 diabetes as an adult.

Can I breast-feed my baby?

Yes. Breast-feeding provides many benefits to your baby. In addition, it may help you lose some of the weight you gained during your pregnancy.

Be aware that blood sugar levels drop while you're breast-feeding, and your baby's bedtime and late-night feedings may deplete your sugar supply. So you may have to adjust your insulin dose, particularly overnight. Your doctor or a diabetes educator can help you adjust your insulin regimen to allow for breast-feeding.

How do I know if my impotence is due to physical or psychological factors?

A sudden inability to maintain an erection is usually related to psychological factors, such as stress. In addition, if you still experience erections while you sleep, your impotence is probably due to psychological factors. A gradual loss of erection, on the other hand, is more likely to be related to physical factors, such as nerve and blood vessel disease.

If the cause of your impotence is uncertain, various tests can help identify its source.

Are treatments for impotence covered by Medicare or private insurance?

Most are, but you may have to pay a portion of the cost yourself, especially for medications.

Additional Resources

Contact these organizations for more information about diabetes. Some groups offer free printed material or videotapes. Others have material or videos you can purchase.

American Association of Diabetes Educators

100 W. Monroe St.
Suite 400
Chicago, IL 60603-1901
312-424-2426
Fax: 312-424-2427
Web site: *www.aadenet.org*

American Diabetes Association

1701 N. Beauregard St.
Alexandria, VA 22311
800-342-2383 (800-DIABETES)
Web site: *www.diabetes.org*

Canadian Diabetes Association

15 Toronto St.
Suite 800
Toronto, ON M5C 2E3
416-363-3373 or 800-226-8464 (800-BANTING)
Web site: *www.diabetes.ca*

Centers for Disease Control and Prevention

1600 Clifton Road
Atlanta, GA 30333
404-639-3534 or 800-311-3435
Web site: *www.cdc.gov*

International Diabetic Athletes Association
1647 W. Bethany Home Road, #B
Phoenix, AZ 85015
800-898-4322 (800-898-IDAA)
Fax: 602-433-9331
Web site: *www.diabetes-exercise.org*

Juvenile Diabetes Foundation International
120 Wall St., 19th floor
New York, NY 10005
212-785-9500 or 800-533-2873 (800-JDF-CURE)
Fax: 212-785-9595
Web site: *www.jdf.org*

Mayo Clinic Health Information
Web site: *www.MayoClinic.com*

National Diabetes Education Initiative
Web site: *www.ndei.org*

National Diabetes Information Clearinghouse
1 Information Way
Bethesda, MD 20892-3560
301-654-3327
Fax: 301-907-8906
Web site: *www.niddk.nih.gov/health/diabetes/ndic.htm*

National Institute of Diabetes and Digestive and Kidney Diseases
Office of Communications and Public Liaison
NIDDK, National Institutes of Health
31 Center Drive, MSC 2560
Bethesda, MD 20892-2560
301-496-3583 or 800-438-5383
Web site: *www.niddk.nih.gov*

Index

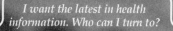

I want the latest in health information. Who can I turn to?

A question of health? Mayo Clinic books are the answer.™

MAYO CLINIC ON HEALTHY WEIGHT

Answers to help you achieve and maintain the weight that's right for you

COMPLETELY REVISED AND UPDATED

MAYO CLINIC FAMILY HEALTH BOOK

THE ULTIMATE ILLUSTRATED HOME MEDICAL REFERENCE

THE Mayo Clinic Williams-Sonoma COOKBOOK

mayo

Questions about health? More and more people are looking to Mayo Clinic for expert, easy-to-understand answers. With an award-winning library of health information resources — including a Web site, books and newsletters — reliable answers to your health questions can be right at your fingertips.

www.MayoClinic.com

© 2001, Mayo Foundation for Medical Education and Research.

When you purchase Mayo Clinic newsletters and books, proceeds are used to further medical education and research at Mayo Clinic. You not only get solutions to your questions on health, but you become part of the answer.

Get answers with these best selling books from Mayo Clinic!

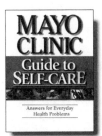
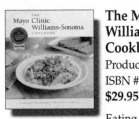
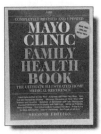
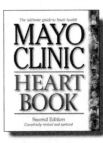

This series of books from Mayo Clinic has answers you're looking for!

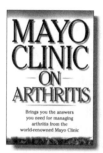

Mayo Clinic on Arthritis
Product # 268500
ISBN # 1-893005-00-3
$14.95

Mayo Clinic on Arthritis provides reliable answers about the most common forms of arthritis — osteo-arthritis and rheumatoid arthritis — with an emphasis on what you can do to manage these conditions. *Mayo Clinic on Arthritis* is recommended by the Arthritis Foundation.

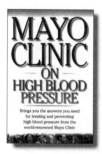

Mayo Clinic on High Blood Pressure
Product # 268400
ISBN # 1-893005-01-1
$14.95

Mayo Clinic on High Blood Pressure provides answers to help you manage high blood pressure. Solutions for controlling your weight, becoming more physically active and eating well are presented realistically, reasonably and reliably. In addition, the book examines the role of medication — when it's necessary and the types available.

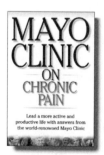

Mayo Clinic on Chronic Pain
Product # 268700
ISBN # 1-893005-02-X
$14.95

An estimated 50 million Americans live with chronic pain. This clearly written book focuses on what you can do to manage long-standing or recurrent pain, from the more familiar headaches, back pain and arthritis to less common and unknown causes.

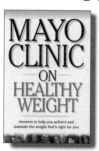

Mayo Clinic on Healthy Weight
Product # 270200
ISBN # 1-893005-05-4
$14.95

Mayo Clinic on Healthy Weight offers sound advice on determining, achieving and maintaining a weight that's healthy for you. It addresses proper nutrition, exercise and other factors that affect weight. You'll find a 16-page color section including recipes, photos and the new Mayo Clinic Healthy Weight Pyramid, a vital component to permanent weight management.

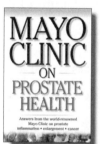

Mayo Clinic on Prostate Health
Product # 268800
ISBN # 1-893005-03-8
$14.95

Whether you or someone you care about has a prostate condition, this book will have the answers you're looking for. *Mayo Clinic on Prostate Health* focuses on three common conditions: prostatitis, benign prostatic hyperplasia (BPH) and prostate cancer.

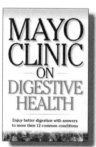

Mayo Clinic on Digestive Health
Product # 268900
ISBN # 1-893005-04-6
$14.95

This book explains a variety of digestive symptoms, including heartburn, abdominal pain, constipation and diarrhea, in plain English. Disorders such as lactose intolerance, GERD, ulcers, irritable bowel syndrome and other digestive problems are discussed.

Available at your favorite bookstore or library, or order direct by calling 800-291-1128. Order code 251.

(Price does not include shipping, handling or applicable sales tax.)

Keep informed . . . with these award-winning monthly publications from Mayo Clinic

The Newsletter Written Especially for Women

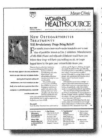 **Mayo Clinic Women's HealthSource** (illustrated)
ISSN # 0091-0880
$27/year (U.S.)
$34/year (Canada)
$42/year (all other countries)

Get your health news from a source you know and trust, Mayo Clinic.

This monthly newsletter is full of reliable, timely information on women's health issues, including treatments, medications, testing and preventive care.

Mayo Clinic draws upon its vast experience in caring for hundreds of thousands of patients to bring you the latest, most accurate, most reliable information available.

Each issue is filled with the important information women need to help them maintain a healthy lifestyle and live their lives to the fullest.

Features:
- 12 issues a year
- 8 pages in each issue
- Full-color medical illustrations
- Accurate, timely and reliable information
- Special monthly feature
- Complete annual index of articles, published by topic

The Leading Health Information Publication

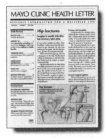 **Mayo Clinic Health Letter** (illustrated)
ISSN # 0741-6245
$27/year (U.S.)
$34/year (Canada)
$42/year (all other countries)

Each issue provides up-to-date, reliable information to help you avoid disease and stay well.

From everyday health matters to serious diseases, this newsletter provides medically accurate answers.

Each issue is written in easy-to-understand language. Even the most complicated medical issues are clearly explained. Every issue contains full-color medical illustrations to aid in learning and comprehension.

Your subscription includes 3 bonus medical essays published throughout the year, each bringing you in-depth coverage of an important health issue that may affect your life.

Features:
- 12 issues a year
- 8 pages in each issue
- Full-color medical illustrations
- Accurate, timely and reliable information
- Three special medical essays
- Complete 3-year index of articles, published by topic

Order newsletters today by calling 800-333-9037.